Atkins Diet Recipes Under 30 Minutes!

Over 30 Atkins Diet Recipes For All Phases (Including Atkins Induction Recipes)

JENNIFER JENKINS

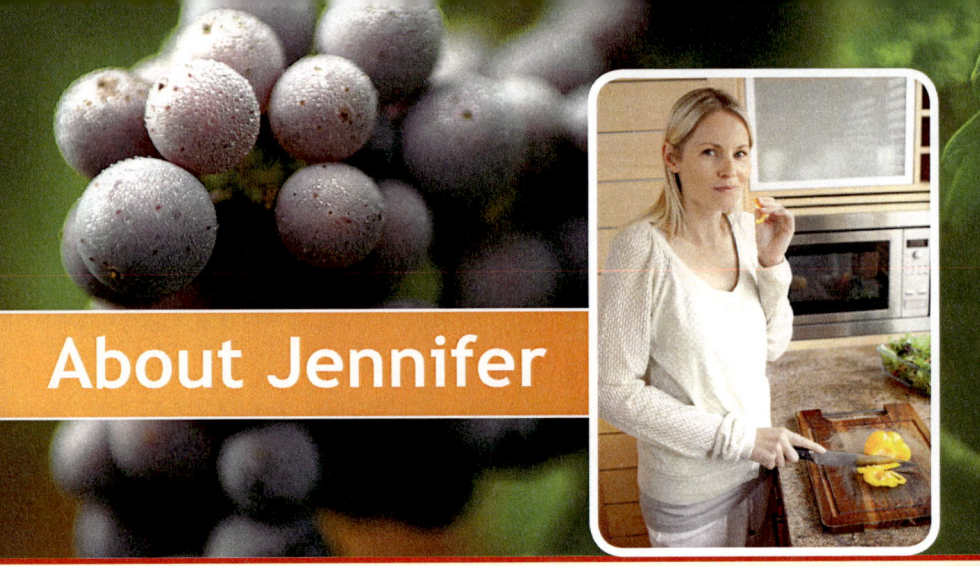

About Jennifer

After failing multiple times to lose weight with the many (often confusing) diets available, Jennifer was at a loss not being able to find a proven diet that works.

This forced her on a two-month long journey as she tried countless methods from joining expensive (and intensive) gym programs, to starving herself for days.

And all thanks to the recipes and techniques shared in her guides, Jennifer's dream of losing 10 pounds safely and naturally was realized… and you can do the same too!

Other Books by Jennifer

High Protein Low Carb Diet - Lose Weight Effortlessly & Permanently

The Ultimate HCG Diet - Safely Lose As Much As One Pound In A Single Day!

The Ultimate Juice Diet - Includes 34 Juicing Recipes for Weight Loss, Detox, Higher Energy and More!

50 Green Smoothie Recipes - For Detox, Weight Loss, Boosting Your Energy & Improving Your Immunity!

Full List: www.amazon.com/author/jenniferjenkins

Table of Contents

Legal & Disclaimer

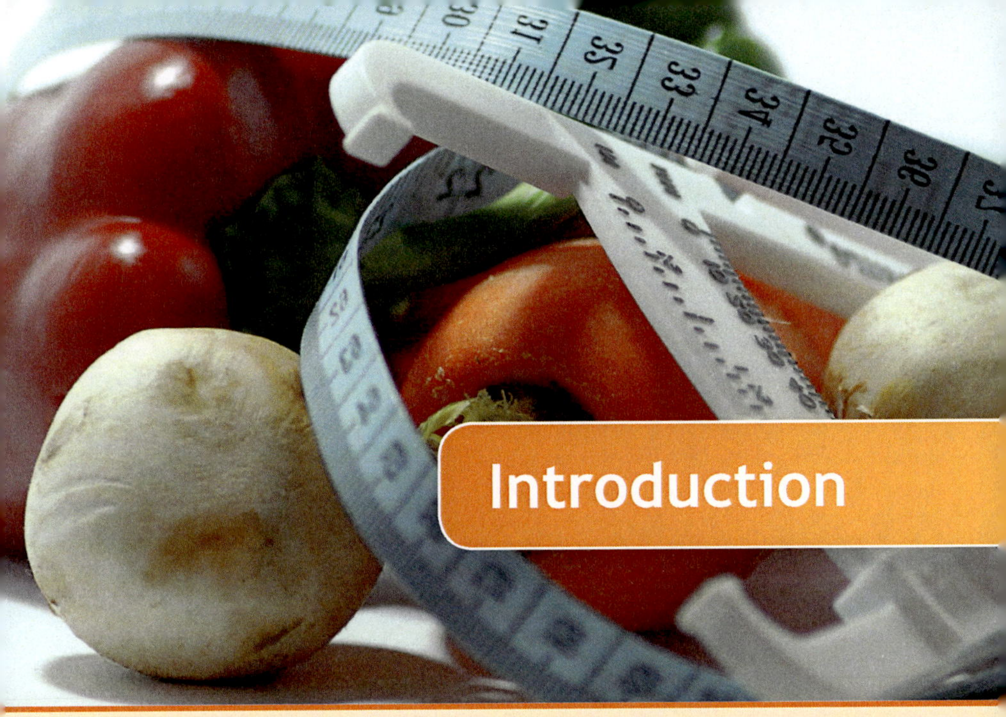

Introduction

The Atkins Diet is by far the most popular diet in the world. If you're like most people who want to shed some weight and live a healthier lifestyle, you've probably heard of it before.

So why is the Atkins Diet so popular? Simply because it also allows you eat red meat, butter, cheese, and eggs --

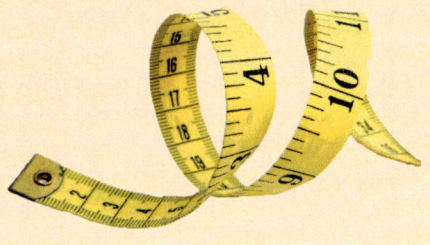

all of which would be considered "prohibited" if you follow other diet plans that focus on lowering fat. But the good news is that these foods take longer for the stomach to digest, so they keep you feeling full for a longer period of time while reducing or even eliminating any hunger pangs! (Who says you need to feel starved when you're dieting?!)

Because of the flexibility in the food you can eat, many people have found the Atkins Diet much more flexible than all other diets in existence. There's no need for you to give up your favorite high fat and protein foods. Even butter, red meat, and mayonnaise are all okay to eat on this diet.

And most importantly, the biggest reason why the Atkins Diet is popular is simply because it works!

According to studies done in 2002 by American Heart Association, the National Institutes of Health, and the Philadelphia Veterans Administration, it has been concluded that low-carbohydrate diets like the Atkins diet are effective in producing faster and more efficient weight-loss results as compared to the weight-loss results with other diet plans.

So Why Does the Atkins Diet Work So Well?

The Atkins Diet follows a 4-phase process that limits your carbohydrate intake and encourages a higher protein intake. Following this diet will send your body into a state of ketoacidosis which in turn leads to:

1. Your body safely and naturally burning its own fats for fuel instead of carbohydrates – it's true! Fat deposits found on the hips, thighs, and abdomen will undergo a natural weight loss through this process, and in time, this will lead to significant weight loss and a healthier, trimmer body.
2. You feeling less hungry for a longer period of time (like I said … you won't go hungry with Atkins!)

Dr. Robert CUP Atkins, a cardiologist, developed the diet in 1974. It is formally known as the Atkins Nutritional Approach which he used to lose his own extra weight.

Before this diet came into fruition, weight loss was largely believed to be achieved solely through limiting your calorie consumption. The Atkins diet revolutionized a different means of thinking by focusing only on limiting your carbohydrate intake.

So … what's the limit for carbohydrate intake per day? The answer: 20 grams. (Don't worry if that sounds low because all the recipes included in this guide are very low in carbohydrates!)

Apart from this somewhat strict restriction, intake of all other food nutrients is not a problem. For example, you can have regular cheese instead of "diet" or "low-fat" cheese, enjoy mayo with your tuna, and even put olive oil on your salads.

Do you like what you're reading so far about the Atkins diet? Then let's continue …

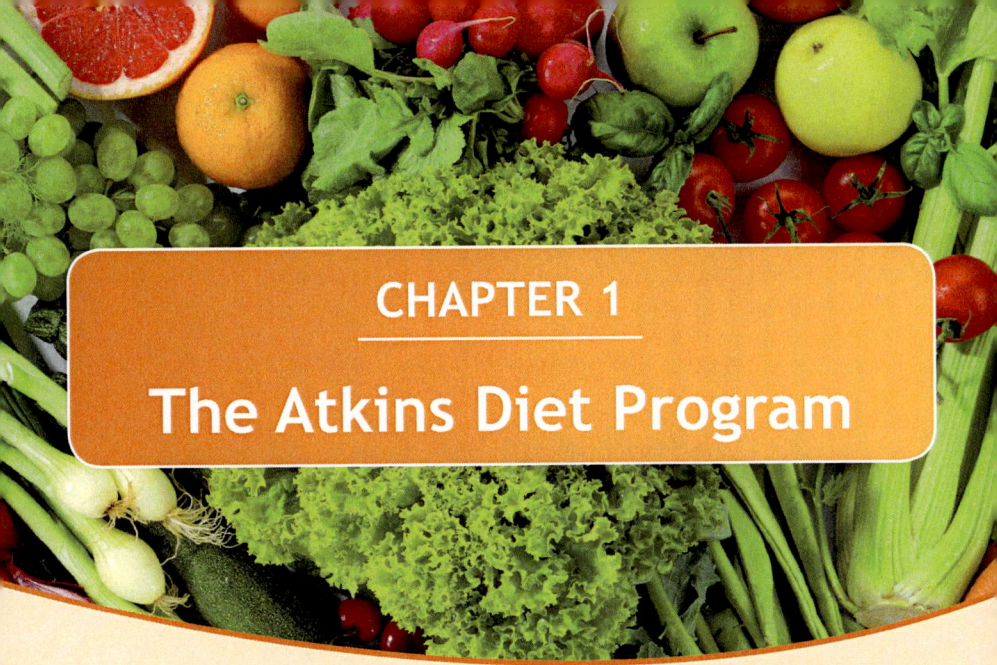

CHAPTER 1

The Atkins Diet Program

The Atkins Diet Program is divided into 4 different phases. Each phase is design to help you ease into the new diet regimen while addressing and improving different areas of your health. This progression will help you achieve your desired results and will encourage dedication to the longevity of the program for a healthier new you for the long haul.

Phase 1: The Induction Phase

This is the first phase of the Atkins Diet, and it is the most restrictive phase out of all 4 phases of the diet. Focusing on the induction phase will send your body into a state of ketosis. Reports of significant weight loss between 5-10 pounds a week is common and has been reported many times.

During this 2-week phase, a carbohydrate intake of up to 20 grams daily is recommended. Dieters can monitor whether they are entering a state of ketosis or not by testing with Ketostix. These should be available at your local pharmacy, but if you don't see them on the shelf, just ask your pharmacist. In addition to using Ketostix, dieters may notice a metallic taste in the mouth or a sweet smell of ketones coming from the breath, sweat, and skin – all indicators of ketosis.

Lose Up To 15 Pounds in Two Weeks

It is during this first phase that you will lose the most weight. The primary focus of Phase 1 is to help you get a jump start on shedding excess pounds! Phase 1 helps you achieve this result by allowing 4-6 ounces of eggs, poultry, fowl, fish, shellfish, or meats, 4 ounces of cheese, leafy greens, and most vegetable oils during each meal. Water intake is very important, and it is vital you drink at least 8 glasses of water daily.

Caffeine is allowed but only in moderation. Alcohol is strictly prohibited.

What You Can Eat During the Induction Phase

Fish:

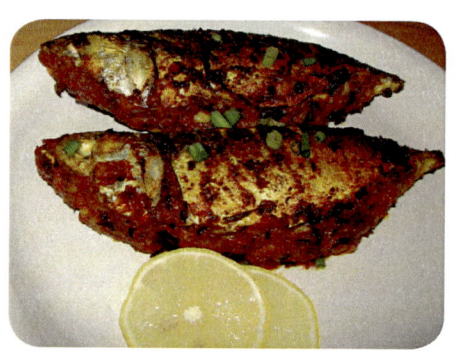

- Halibut
- Cod
- Herring
- Flounder
- Trout
- Tuna
- Sole
- Sardines
- Salmon

Fowl:

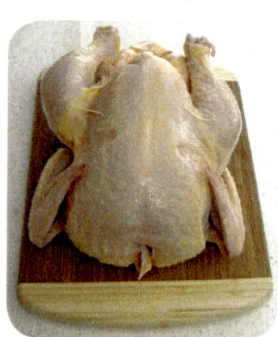

- Ostrich
- Turkey
- Quail
- Goose
- Pheasant
- Duck
- Cornish Hen
- Chicken

Shellfish:

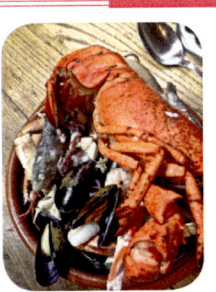

- • Squid
- • Shrimp
- • Lobster
- • Mussels
- • Clams
- • Crabmeat

Other Meats:

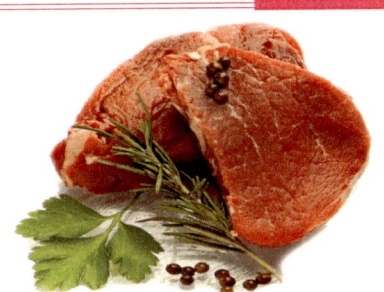

- Lamb
- Ham
- Beef
- Venison
- Veal
- Bacon

Miscellaneous:

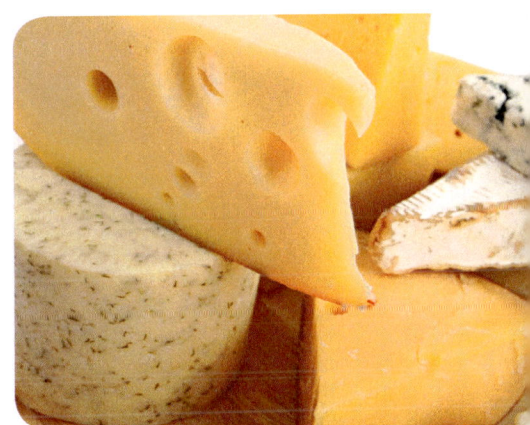

- Eggs
- Cheese (3-4 ounces daily)
- Vegetables (more or less 1 cup or 12-15 grams which depends on the carbohydrate content of the vegetable chosen)
- Herbs
- Mayonnaise (with no added sugar)
- Butter
- Vegetable oils
- Olive oil
- Clear broth
- Herbal tea
- Water

TIPS

1. Small, frequent meals spaced out to 4-5 meals a day are recommended. Regular meals of 3 times daily are also allowed. Never keep yourself from eating for more than 6 hours at a time.
2. Include at least 4-6 ounces of protein in your diet each day. Use a variety of vegetable proteins, or meats such as shellfish, veal, pork, lamb, or beef. Trimming excess fat off the meat is not necessary, but if you choose to do so, replace it with a splash of olive oil instead.
3. Aim for 1 tablespoon of oil on your salads choosing from canola, olive, or safflower oils. Butter, nut oils, and mayonnaise can also be consumed.
4. Refrain from ricotta or cottage cheese, but most other cheeses are fine – just aim for a daily limit of 4 ounces per day. Green olives are limited to 10-20 pieces. Take care to limit yourself to half an avocado, 3 tablespoons of lime or lemon juice, and 2-3 tablespoons of cream. When using artificial sweeteners, strive not to go beyond using 3 packs a day. Sugar-free desserts are a great alternative to tame your sweet tooth.
5. Consume 8 glasses of water and other approved beverages such as herbal teas or club soda each day. Soups or broth can be consumed as well. Limit the intake of caffeine and definitely avoid alcohol during this time.
6. Take supplements like omega-3 or iron-free multivitamins.
7. Never skimp on fat intake or make yourself hungry.
8. Be on the lookout for hidden carbohydrates when eating out. These can often be found in gravy or salad dressings.

10 Induction Phase Recipes

Garlic Lime Chicken

Ingredients:

- ¾ teaspoon salt
- ¼ teaspoon dried parsley
- ¼ teaspoon thyme
- ½ teaspoon garlic powder
- ¼ teaspoon onion powder
- ¼ teaspoon cayenne
- ⅛ teaspoon cayenne

- ¼ teaspoon black pepper
- Boneless chicken breasts, 6 pieces
- Lime juice, 3 tablespoons
- Olive oil, 1 tablespoons
- Garlic powder, 2 teaspoons
- Butter, 2 teaspoons

Preparation:

1. Mix the first 7 spices together.
2. Coat chicken with the spice mixture.
3. Place the butter and oil in the skillet over medium heat.
4. Sauté the chicken breasts until they are golden brown in color.
5. Using the remaining garlic powder and lime juice to season the chicken pieces.
6. Coat evenly while sautéing.

Nutritional Information:

- Calories-320
- Fat-9g
- Protein-55g
- Carbohydrates-2g
- Sodium-460mg

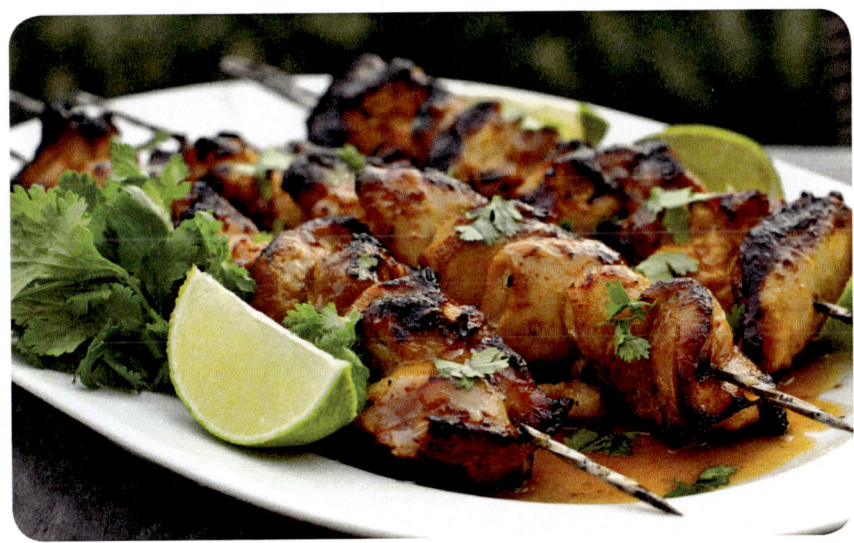

Creamy Chicken and Mushrooms

Ingredients:

- Vegetable oil, 1 teaspoon
- Garlic, 2 cloves – crushed
- Bacon, 2 slices – chopped
- Chicken, 1 cup of sliced lean meat
- Mixed mushrooms, 12 ounce
- Cream, 1 cup
- Chicken stock, ½ cup
- Brandy, 2 ounce
- Black pepper

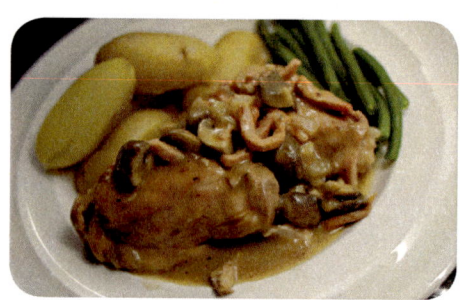

Preparation:

1. Heat oil in a wok over medium heat.
2. Add bacon and garlic then stir-fry until bacon turns golden brown.
3. Add the chicken and continue stir-frying until chicken becomes tender.
4. Set aside the chicken in a separate container and keep warm.
5. Using the same wok, fry mushrooms and spring onions until tender.
6. Add the chicken back in and continue to stir-fry for 5 more minutes.
7. Add the brandy, stock, and cream then bring to a boil.
8. Lower heat and allow the dish to simmer until the sauce decreases by half.
9. Season with black pepper.

Nutritional Information:

- Calories-387
- Fat-22g
- Proten-32g
- Carbohydrates-8g
- Dietary Fiber-1g
- Cholesterol-123mg
- Sodium-423mg
- Serves 4

French Chicken Provençale

Ingredients:

- Chicken breast, 4 slices
- Olive oil, ¼ cup
- Garlic, 2 cloves – minced
- Fresh mushrooms, 4 ounces
- Onions, ½ cup – chopped
- Bacon, 4 slices – chopped
- Butter, 2 tablespoons
- 1 small Bay leaf
- Dried thyme, ¼ teaspoon
- Dry white wine, ¼ cup
- Chicken broth or water, 1½ cup
- Green bell pepper, ½ cup – cut into strips
- Plum tomatoes, 4 pieces – cut into large wedges.

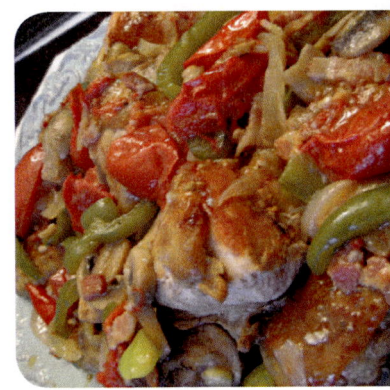

Preparation:

1. Brown the chicken in oil in a skillet then remove and set aside.
2. Brown the other ingredients listed above in the skillet that still has the drippings from the cooked chicken.
3. Add all the ingredients to a pot, pour the broth over them, and then simmer for 40 minutes over low heat.
4. Once the chicken is done and the vegetables are tender, you can thicken the broth with tomato sauce.
5. Cook only until the tomatoes are soft but intact and the green peppers have barely gone limp.

Nutritional Information:

- Calories-504
- Fat-33.3g
- Carbs-8g
- Fiber-1.9g
- Protein-40g
- Serves 4

Tuna Swiss Quiche

Ingredients:

- Tuna, 2 cans – drained
- Swiss cheese, 1 cup – shredded
- Half and half, 1 cup
- Mayonnaise, 1 cup
- Onions, ½ cup – chopped
- 3 eggs

Preparation:

1. Mix everything together and pour into a pie pan after spraying with non-stick spray.
2. Bake in a 350 degree oven for 50 minutes.

Nutritional Information:

- Calories-490g
- Fat-41.6g
- Carbohydrates-4.8g
- Protein-24.16g

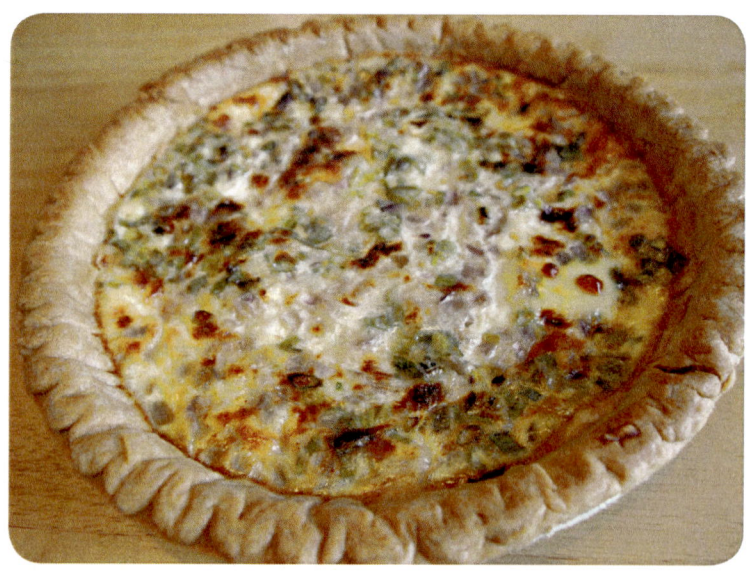

Bacon and Leek Soup

Ingredients:

- Low-sodium Bacon, 5 slices
- Leeks, 2 pieces – washed and thinly sliced
- Salt and pepper to taste
- Heavy cream, 2 cups
- Water, 2 cups
- Homemade chicken broth, 2 cups
- Your favorite thickener (optional)

Preparation:

1. In a large pot, brown the bacon.
2. Add the sliced leeks.
3. As soon as the leeks begin to wilt, add in the water, chicken stock, salt, and pepper.
4. Allow to simmer for a few minutes in order to incorporate all the flavors.
5. Add in the cream.
6. Add a thickener (such as a little cornstarch or flour) if a thicker consistency is desired.

Nutritional Information:

- Calories-377g
- Fat-37 g
- Carbs-5.58g
- Protein-6.1g
- Sodium-211g
- Potassium-216g

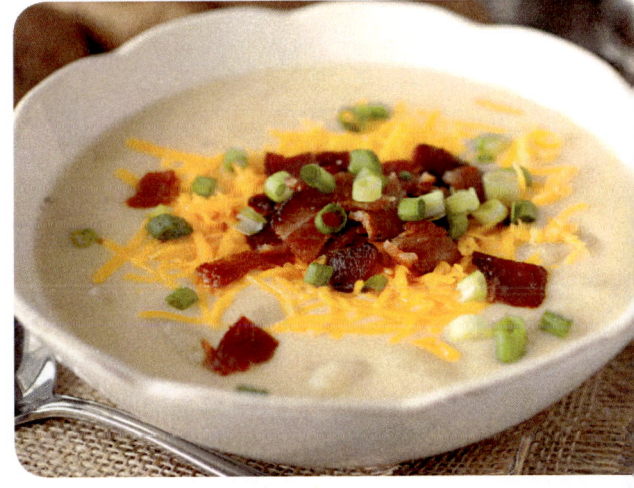

Meatballs Stroganoff

Ingredients:

- Ground beef, 1 pound
- Parmesan cheese, 3 tablespoons – grated
- Onion, 2 tablespoon – minced
- 1 Egg
- Salt and pepper to taste
- Garlic, 1 clove
- Dried parsley, 1 teaspoon
- Olive oil, 1 teaspoon
- Sour cream, ¼ cup
- Beef broth, 8 ounces
- Low carb thickener, 1 teaspoon

Preparation:

1. Mix together the first 8 ingredients.
2. Form into meatballs.
3. Brown the meatballs in the olive oil in a large pan.
4. Pour off the oil and set aside.
5. Add in beef broth and sour cream.
6. If using a thickener, add it in now.
7. Allow to simmer on low heat until sauce is reduced by half.

Nutritional Information:

- Calories-379g
- Carbs-2.97g
- Protein-31.9g
- Fat-26.54g

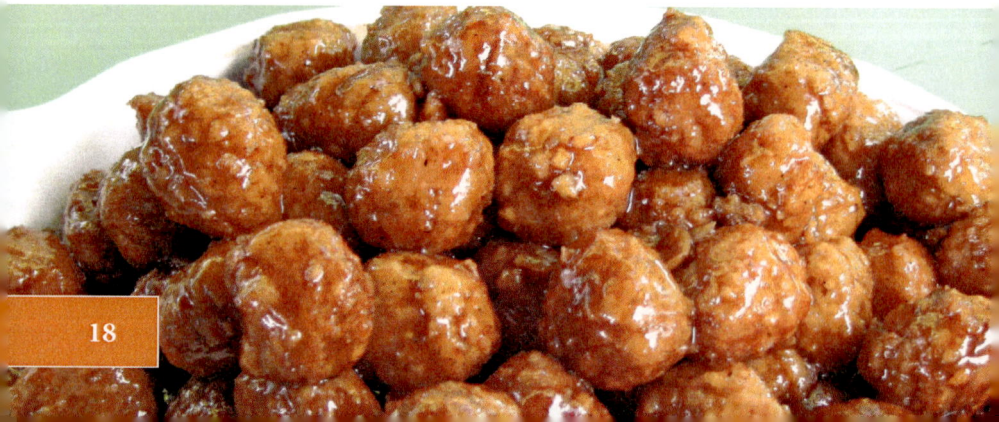

Beef Bok Choy

Ingredients:

- Coconut oil, 2 tablespoons
- Onion, 2 ounces – sliced
- Beef, 1 pounds – thinly sliced
- Bok Choy, 2 stalks – washed and sliced
- Mushrooms, 6 medium sized – sliced
- Red bell pepper, 2 ounces – diced
- Ginger, 1 teaspoon – minced
- Garlic, 2 cloves – minced
- Hoisin sauce, 3 tablespoons
- Chile paste, ½ teaspoon
- Low-sodium soy sauce, 1 tablespoon

Preparation:

1. Heat a large skillet then add the oils.
2. Once they are hot, add the onion and sauté.
3. Add the beef next and sear until it is no longer pink.
4. Place all other vegetables, garlic, and ginger (except bok choy).
5. Once the veggies are tender but still crisp, add in the bok choy.
6. Add the beef broth and the remaining ingredients.

Nutritional Information:

- Calories-281.3g
- Fat-15.5
- Carbs-7.73g
- Protein-27.7g
- Sodium-512g
- Potassium-881g

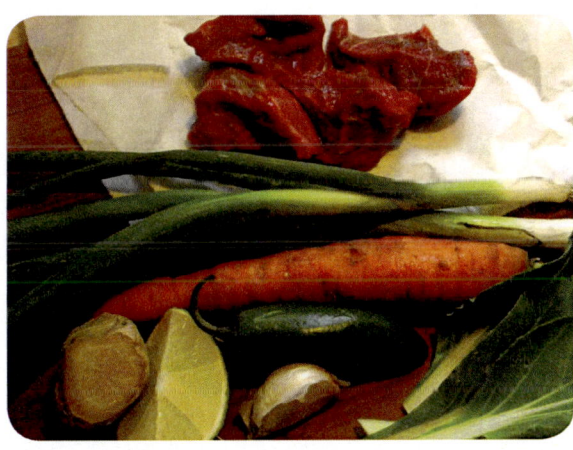

Sausage Hash

Ingredients:

- Lean homemade pork sausage, 6 ounces
- Onion, 2 ounces – chopped
- Bacon grease, 1 tablespoon
- Radishes, 1 cup – cubed
- Smoked Gouda cheese, 2 ounces – shredded

Preparation:

1. Place bacon grease in a skillet over high heat.
2. Add the onion and sauté until it starts to caramelize.
3. Add the sausage and then brown well.
4. Add in the radishes and continue to sauté until they become tender.
5. Place on a serving plate and top with cheese.
6. Place in a microwave or under a hot broiler until the cheese is just melted. Serve.

Nutritional Information:

- Calories-465
- Fat-39g
- Carbs-5.1g
- Fiber-1.2g
- Protein-23.2g
- Potassium-418g
- Sodium-1050

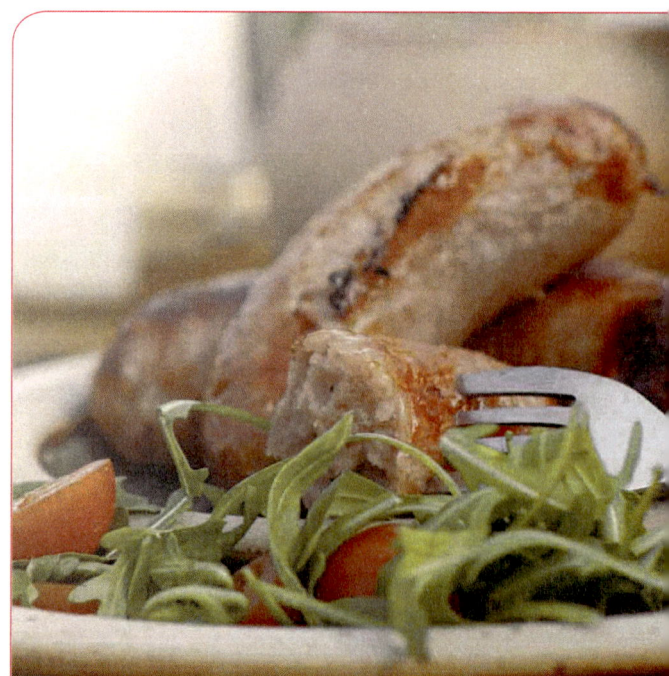

Bacon Pork Patties

Ingredients:

- Lean ground pork, 1 pound
- 1 Egg – beaten
- Onion, 1 ½ ounces – finely minced
- Celery, 1/3 cup – finely chopped
- Bacon, 4 ounces – finely chopped
- Lemon pepper, ¾ teaspoon
- Dash of poultry seasoning
- Dash of black pepper
- Chopped parsley, 3 tablespoons – finely chopped

Preparation:

1. Bacon brown slightly in a large skillet over medium heat.
2. Add in the celery and onion then sauté until tender.
3. Spoon the veggies into a bowl.
4. Add the rest of the ingredients to the vegetable/bacon mixture and combine thoroughly.
5. Divide into 4 equal portions then flatten into meat patties.
6. Once the patties are formed, brown them in a skillet until golden brown on each side.
7. Serve with your favorite sauce.

Nutritional Information:

Calories-452
Fat-38g
Carbs-1.5g
Protein-28.2g
Sodium-325mg
Potassium-440mg

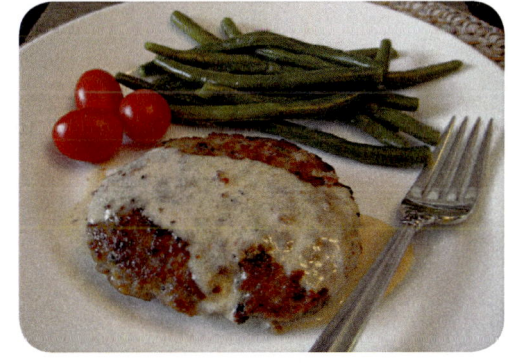

Thai Chicken Soup

Ingredients:

- Cooked chicken, 12 ounces – shredded or cut up
- Onion, 4 ounces – chopped
- Red bell pepper, ½ cup – chopped
- Garlic, 1 clove – minced
- 1 Carrot – sliced
- 3 Green cabbages – chopped
- Ginger root, 1 teaspoon – peeled and minced
- Coconut cream, 1 cup
- Chicken broth, 4 cups
- Toasted sesame seeds, 1 tablespoon
- Thai red curry paste, 2 tablespoons
- Black sesame seeds, 1 tablespoon
- Sesame oil, 1 teaspoon

Preparation:

1. In a large pot, mix all ingredients except for sesame oil and coconut cream.
2. Bring to a boil over high heat.
3. Reduce to a simmer for about 20 minutes.
4. Once carrots are tender, add coconut cream.
5. Simmer for another 2-3 minutes.
6. Just before serving, add sesame oil, and sprinkle sesame seeds on top.

Nutritional Information:

- Calories-315
- Fat-20.3g
- Carbs-11.5g
- Protein-27.4g
- Sodium-325mg
- Potassium-593mg

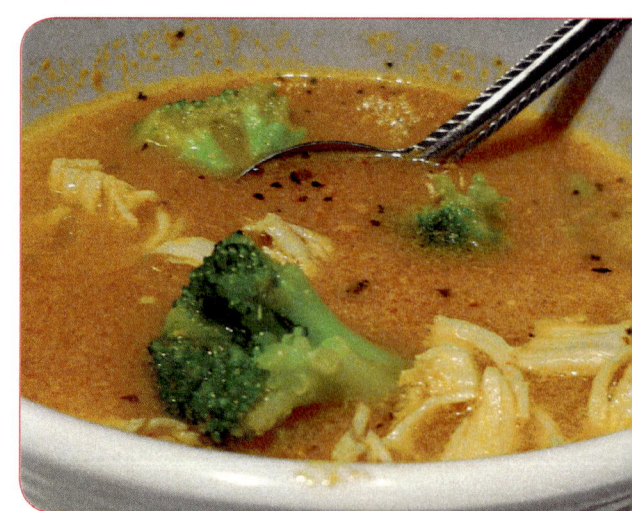

Phase 2: On-Going Weight Loss (OWL)

In the second phase of the Atkins Diet, your carbohydrate intake will gradually increase 5 grams each week. During this ongoing phase, your goal is to find your individually unique "Critical Carbohydrate Level for Losing". You are allowed to increase your carbohydrate intake each week for 3 weeks until you stop losing weight or when you are about 10 pounds away from your goal weight.

Lose Weight – Slowly and Safely

For the first week, you begin by increasing your carbohydrate intake to 25 grams daily. The following week you will add another 5 grams. This means that by week 2 you should be consuming 30 grams of carbohydrates per day. You then continue with this phase until your body stops losing weight. When this happens, subtract 5 grams from the current carbohydrate intake amount, and maintain that level for the rest of your time on the Atkins Diet.

What You Can Eat During the OWL Phase

- Nuts and Seeds
- Cheese
- Alcohol
- Berries
- Whole Grains
- Starchy Vegetables
- Fruit
- Lime Juice
- Lemon Juice
- Tomato Juice
- Ricotta Cheese
- Mozzarella Cheese
- Heavy Cream

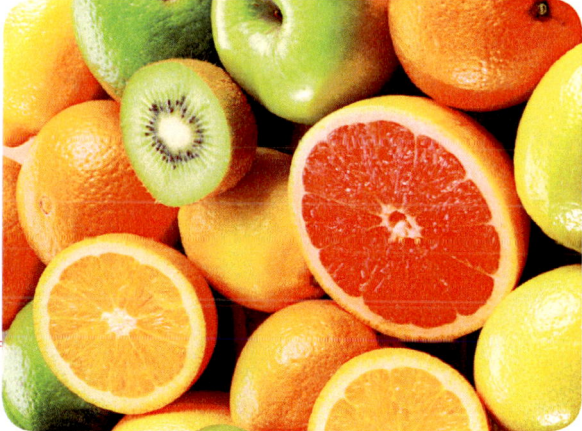

TIPS

1. Weight loss during the OWL phase slows down to 1-2 pounds a week. You focus on increasing your carbohydrate intake until you are no longer losing weight in order to find the perfect balance for your body.
2. Strictly avoid simple carbohydrates such as cakes, cookies, pastries, white bread, white rice, and refined pasta.
3. Rotate carbohydrates around vegetables, nuts and seeds, cheese, legumes, alcohol, whole grains, certain fruits, and alcohol.
4. Continue drinking at least 8 glasses of water per day.
5. While your body is losing weight, it is vital to continuously replace salt loss. Some foods high in sodium are broths, tomatoes, cheese, and pickles.
6. This second phase is a slow process, so you should not rush into the next stage (Phase 3) too quickly.

Phase 3: Pre-Maintenance

During this phase your goal is to find your personal "Critical Carbohydrate Level for Maintenance". Simply put, this is the maximum level of carbohydrates intake you can consume each day without putting on weight. During this stage your body will begin to get used to your new and healthy way of eating. You will lose fat on your own, and ketosis will stop doing the weight loss work for you.

Maintain Your Control and Your Weight

Think of this stage as a training ground for your body to get used to the low-carbohydrate diet you will be maintaining for the rest of your life. Adding "forbidden carbs" during this time is allowed, but only in strict moderation. This is when your body's protection against ketosis slows down since it is preparing for long-term maintenance.

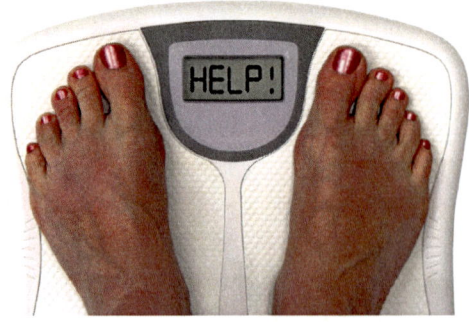

Once you're able to reach your goal weight, maintain at that level for a month or two. You can then increase daily carb consumption by another 10 grams to see if it is possible to do so without gaining any weight. If you notice you've started gaining weight at this level, reduce your carbohydrate level by 5 grams. Do this until you find your tipping point, and then stick with the carbohydrate level that works for your body.

What You Can Eat During Pre-Maintenance

- Yams
- Potatos
- Carrots
- Acorn Squash
- Chickpeas
- Great Northern Beans
- Black Beans
- Lima Beans
- Navy Beans
- Lentils
- Kidney Beans

- Apples
- Bananas
- Watermelon
- Plums
- Peaches
- Guava
- Grapes
- Kiwis
- Cherries
- Rice
- Oatmeal

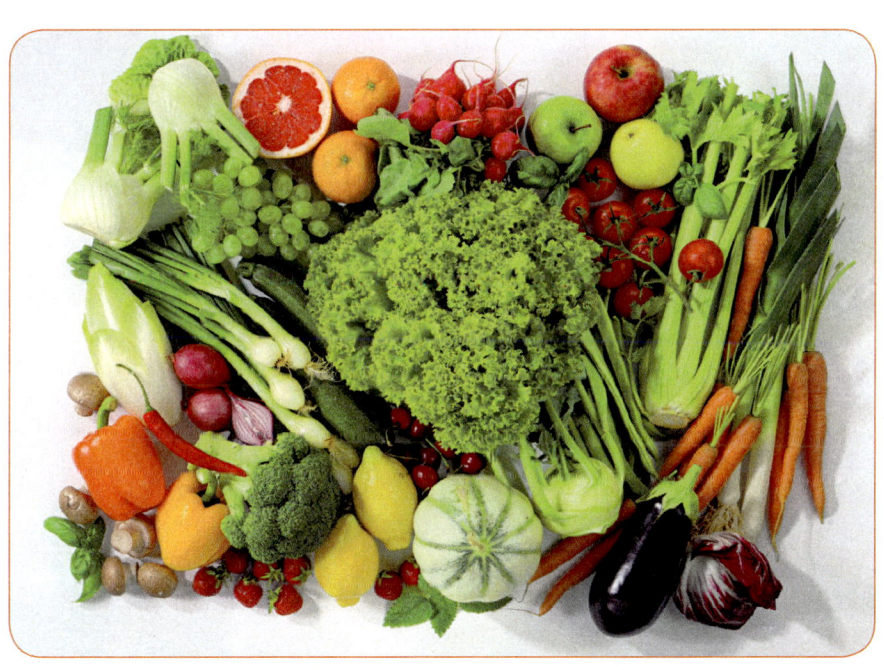

TIPS

1. As with the previous phases, avoidance of sweets, refined foods, and other sugary foods is a must.
2. Add approximately 10 grams of carbohydrates to your diet each week. Once the weight loss stops, decrease the current amount by 5 grams. This may take several weeks, but persevere. Stick with what works for you!
3. During this time you can experiment with more carbs. Pair common sources of carbohydrates with legumes such as black beans, lima beans, or pinto beans. Alternatively, a wider variety of starchy foods such as acorn squash, yams, and potatoes are allowed.
4. Add more grains such as oatmeal and rice back into your diet.
5. You can figure out your carbohydrate intake by planning for higher carbohydrate meals. For example, let's say your critical carbohydrate level is 80 grams per day. During your experimental week, you can have only 60 grams a day then increase this to 100 grams the next week. You can expect to have some carbohydrate cravings at this time.
6. Make sure to eat protein along with fats during this time. It can help decrease carbohydrate cravings while helping you avoid gaining weight as well.

Phase 4: Lifetime Maintenance

With the habits learned in the previous phases, you have reached the point where you need to maintain these habits for life. It may be tempting to fall back to old habits once you've reached your goal weight, but that will quickly undo all the hard work you've done. You're at your goal weight by this time, and the only thing for you to do is keep doing what works for you.

Show the World You Can Stick With the Atkins Diet and Lifestyle

Once you have transitioned into this stage, the only thing left for you to do is exercise strict compliance to the diet. If you find yourself reaching for that cupcake, make sure you turn to your diet guidelines instead. But if you find yourself unable to control the cravings and wind up on a holiday carb binge, regain control by reverting back to the induction phase of your diet. Don't worry … as soon as you've grown accustomed to the diet again, you will be find your craving for carbs decreasing.

One good way to keep yourself on track is to join a support group. Look for other Atkins dieters, or even other friends committed to living a healthy lifestyle. Being around people with similar goals will help you continue to work towards achieving your own goals. Another great way to cope during this lifetime phase is to get involved in a regular exercise schedule. It is a great way to strengthen your body and further maintain your weight loss.

What You Can Eat During Lifetime Maintenance

- Legumes
- Starchy Vegetables
- Bananad
- Apples
- Kiwis
- Guavas
- Plums
- Peaches
- Pasta
- Oatmeal
- Rice
- Grapefruit
- Grapes
- All other carbs listed in the previous phases

TIPS

1. Stay focused on your food choices. Remember that the ketosis process in the 1st phase is not applicable anymore.
2. Once you start experiencing cravings, don't automatically reach for the high-carb foods you're craving. Instead, suppress those desires with protein and fat first. If you happen to fall back and give in to these cravings, just return to Phase 1, and start over again.
3. Weigh yourself every week and note any difference indicated by the scales. Examine your diet and figure out the possible reasons for any discrepancies noticed.
4. Consume unprocessed foods for the most part.
5. If you feel better about going under your carbohydrate count, feel free to do so.
6. Stick with a reliable supplement. You should take a good multivitamin rich in zinc, chromium, magnesium, and all other important essential nutrients.
7. Focus your diet primarily around protein, fruits, and vegetables. Limit your intake of cheese, oils, and dairy products.
8. Incorporate exercise into your diet regimen. Start by walking and slowly stretching out your muscles. It can also be very beneficial to join a local gym or exercise program in order to further your weight loss and live a healthier life.

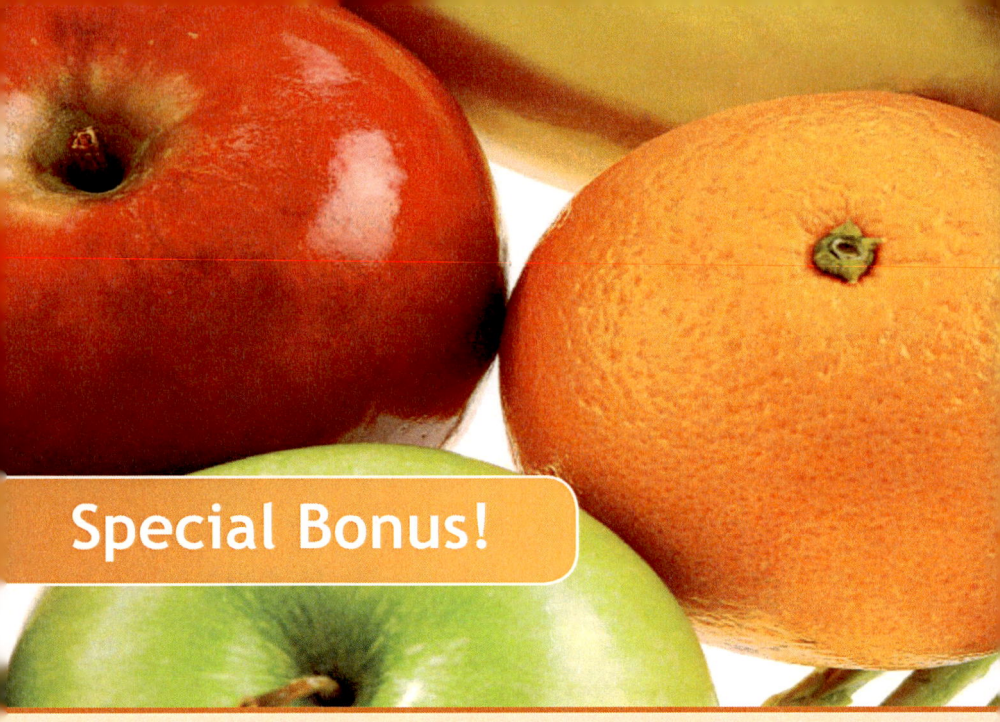

Special Bonus!

Before I continue, I'm really grateful you gave me a chance to help you, so I've specially prepared a 'Bonus Guide' for you to support you in your journey of achieving the dream body or the level of health you've always wanted.

In this guide you'll get *10 Healthy Dinner Recipes* you can prepare easily and quickly. Even children and other picky eaters will enjoy these delicious dinners.

All of these recipes are complete with step-by-step instructions to follow when preparing your next dinner without any fuss or kitchen mess.

This guide is <u>absolutely free</u> to you.

All you have to do is register your email at the URL below so I know where to send the download link:

http://www.expertsfeatured.com/jennifer-bonus-recipes/

CHAPTER 2

Atkins Diet Recipes With 30 Minutes of Cooking Time or Less

In this section, you will find recipes that are very simple and easy to make. You can use these recipes throughout all 4 phases of your Atkins Diet. Enjoy!

10 Recipes for Breakfast

Best Banana Bread

Ingredients:

- 2 mashed bananas
- Coconut flour, 1/3 cup
- Almond flour, 2/3 cup
- Sea salt, ¼ teaspoon
- Glucomannan powder, 1 tablespoon
- Liquefied coconut oil, 3 tablespoons
- Unsalted butter, 1 stick – melted
- Vanilla, ½ teaspoon
- 8 Eggs – beaten

Preparation:

1. Preheat oven to 350 degrees.
2. Using a bit of coconut oil or butter, grease a standard-size loaf pan.
3. Combine dry ingredients in a mixing bowl.
4. Thoroughly mix the wet ingredients in a much larger bowl.
5. Then add in the dry ingredients and whisk until smooth.
6. Fold in fruit or any other nuts you desire.
7. Spoon the mixture into the prepared loaf pan.
8. Bake at 350 degrees for 40-45 minutes or until a toothpick inserted into the center of the loaf comes out clean.

Nutritional Information:

- Calories-141
- Fat-12g
- Carbs-5.6g
- Protein-4.24g
- Sodium-90mg
- Potassium-78mg

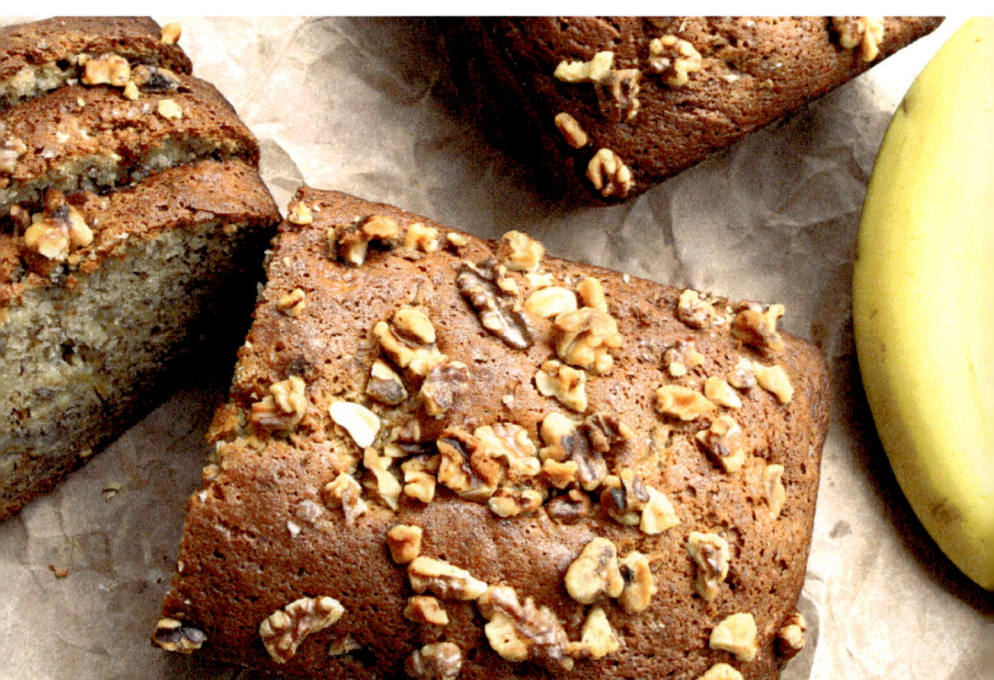

Red Anjou Pear Pancakes

Ingredients:

- 3 Eggs – beaten
- Unsalted butter, 3 tablespoons
- 2 Pears – sliced into ½-inch cubes
- Golden flax meal, ½ cup plus 2 tablespoons
- Coconut cream, 1 tablespoon
- Coconut flour, 2 teaspoons
- Almond flour, 4 tablespoons
- Baking powder, 1 teaspoons
- Cinnamon, ¼ teaspoon
- Maple syrup, 2 tablespoons
- Water (as needed)

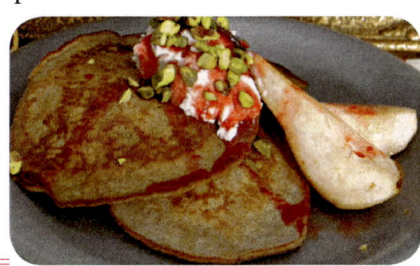

Preparation:

1. Dice the pears into ½" cubes.
2. Melt 1 tablespoon of butter in a large mixing bowl.
3. Then add all the wet ingredients to the bowl along with half of the diced pears.
4. Next, add the dry ingredients to the wet ingredients and mix well.
5. If the batter is too thick, add 1 tablespoon of water at a time until you reach the desired consistency.
6. Melt butter on a non-stick griddle over high heat.
7. Add cinnamon and remaining pear cubes to the batter.
8. Let the butter heat for a few minutes and then reduce heat to low.
9. Pour a scoop of batter onto hot griddle using a measuring cup.
10. Brown and then flip to the other side and continue cooking.
11. Once done, place each pancake on a plate and add the fruit toppings of choice.

Nutritional Information:

- Calories-203.5g
- Fat-16.42g
- Carbs-9.82g
- Protein-6.65g
- Sodium-117mg
- Potassium-155mg

Paleo Eggs Benedict

Ingredients:

- 1 large egg – beaten
- Unsalted butter, ½ tablespoon
- Cauliflower, ½ cup cooked and seasoned
- Sprinkle of cayenne
- **Shawarma dressing:**
- ½ cup mayonnaise
- Ground cumin seed, 2 tablespoons
- Coriander seed, 2 tablespoons
- Turmeric, 2 tablespoons
- Black pepper, 1 tablespoon
- Cayenne, 1 teaspoon
- Garlic powder, 2 teaspoons
- Onion powder, 1 teaspoon
- dash of salt and pepper

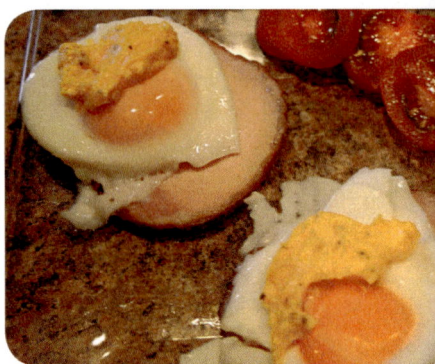

Preparation:

1. Scramble eggs in the usual process in a skillet over medium heat.
2. Place the pre-cooked and re-heated cauliflower on the serving plate.
3. Spoon scrambled eggs on top of the cauliflower.
4. Drizzle with Shawarma dressing and sprinkle cayenne over the top before serving.

Nutritional Information:

- Calories-332g
- Fat-31.3g
- Carbs-4.3g
- Fiber-2.1g
- Protein-10.4g
- Sodium-374mg
- Potassium-213mg

Lemon-Orange Marmalade

Ingredients:

- 4 Meyer lemons
- 1 Naval orange
- EzSweets liquid – sucralose, ¾ teaspoon

Preparation:

1. After washing, cut fruit into smaller pieces and remove as many seeds as possible.
2. Place in food processor and add sweetener.
3. Pulse until it reaches the desired consistency.
4. Place into a clean jar and refrigerate.

Nutritional Information:

- Calories-12.11g
- Fat-.01g
- Carbs-2.5g
- Fiber-0.29g,
- Protein-0.16g

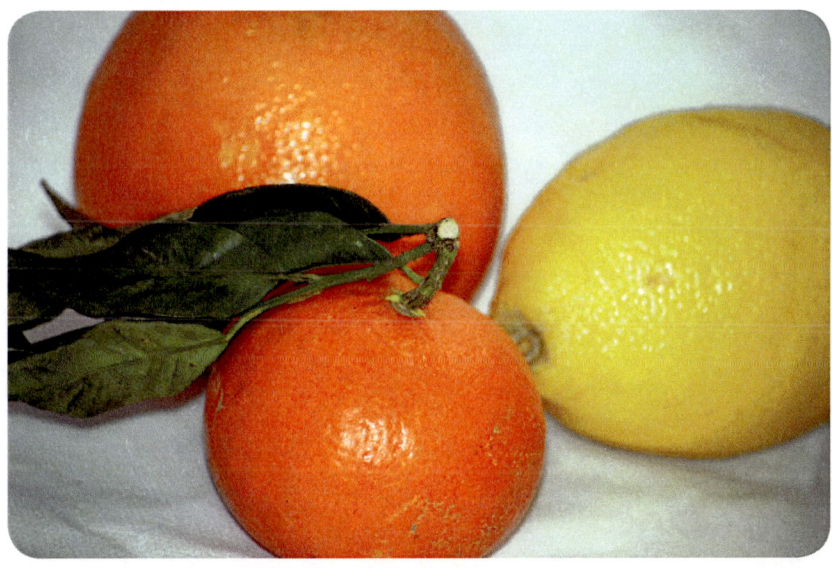

Sausage Tarragon Cream on Toast

Ingredients:

- 1 Roma tomato – chopped
- Green onions, 1/3 cup – chopped
- Heavy cream, ¼ cup
- Water, 1 cup
- Dried tarragon, ¼ teaspoon
- Dash of salt and pepper
- 4 Sausages

Preparation:

1. Brown sausages in a non-stick skillet over medium-high heat.
2. Add green onions and tomato.
3. Sauté until onion begins to soften and tomato is tender but not cooked to mush. Reduce heat to low.
4. Add seasonings, cream, and water.
5. Simmer until thick. Add thickener if desired.

Nutritional Information:

- Calories-330g
- Fat-26.7g
- Carbs-4.3g
- Protein-17.5g
- Potassium-328mg
- Sodium-522mg

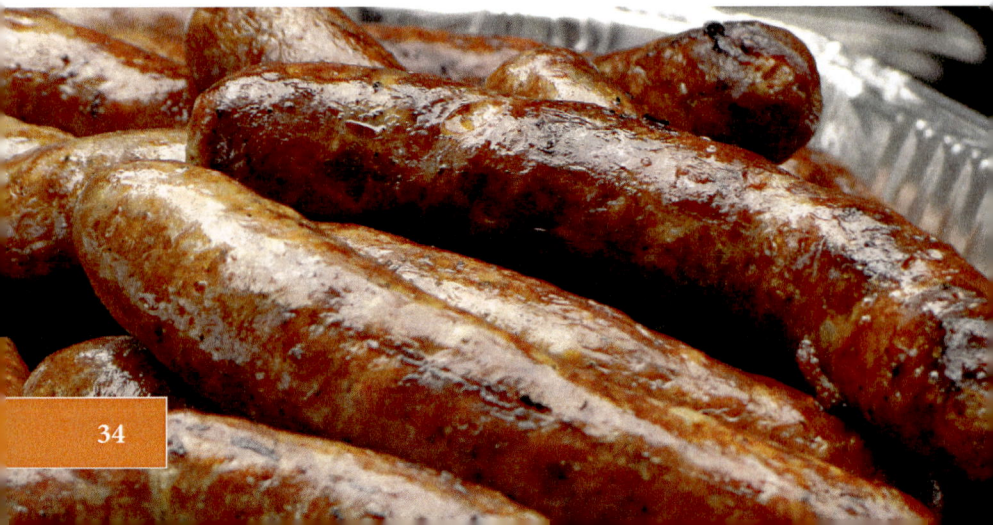

Banana Pancakes

Ingredients:

- Unsalted butter, 1 tablespoon – melted
- 2 eggs – beaten
- Bananas, 3/4 cup – mashed
- Stevia or Splenda, 1 pack
- Flax meal, 1 cup
- Almond flour, 2 tablespoons
- Coconut flour, 2 teaspoons
- Baking powder, 1 teaspoon
- Cinnamon, ¼ teaspoon

Preparation:

1. Melt butter in microwave.
2. Add in bananas and eggs.
3. Next add cream and stir well.
4. Measure and then add all dry ingredients to the egg mixture.
5. Stir well to form batter.
6. If batter is too thick, add a bit of water until desired consistency is reached.
7. Preheat the griddle and grease lightly.
8. Pour around 1/3 cup of batter on hot griddle and brown well on each side. Serve.

Nutritional Information:

- Calories 132.3g
- Fat-9.52g
- Carbs-8.78g
- Protein-4.87g
- Sodium-91.7mg
- Potassium-174mg

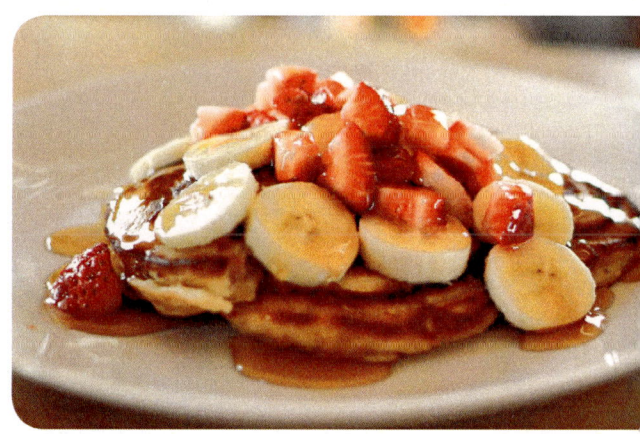

Blackberry Flax Muffins

Ingredients:

- Unsalted butter, 2 tablespoons – melted
- 5 large eggs – beaten
- Liquid Splenda, 2 drops
- Cream, 6 tablespoons
- Blackberries, 1 cup – coarsely chopped
- Stevia, 4-5 packets
- Almond flour, ½ cup
- Cinnamon, ½ teaspoon
- Flax meal, 1 cup
- Oat fiber, 2 tablespoons
- Baking powder, 2 ½ teaspoons

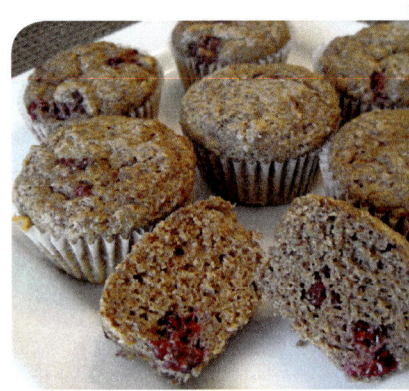

Preparation:

1. Melt butter in microwave.
2. Add in the eggs.
3. Next add cream and liquid Splenda and combine well.
4. Add in the rest of the dry ingredients and stir until mixed.
5. Fold in the berries gently and be careful not to over-mix them.
6. Line and grease muffin tin.
7. Add scoop of batter to each muffin well and allow to bake for 20 minutes or until firm to the touch in the center.

Nutritional Information:

- Calories-183g
- Fat-16g
- Carbs-6.74g
- Protein-5.73g
- Potassium-133mg
- Sodium-140mg

Rutabaga and Onion Hash Browns

Ingredients:

- Onion, 2 ounce – chopped
- Rutabaga, 5 ounces – dried and peeled
- Bacon grease, 1 tablespoon
- Dash of salt and pepper

Preparation:

1. Heat bacon grease in skillet then add and sauté the onions over high heat until halfway done.
2. Add in the rutabaga and turn often until fairly tender. This will take about 15 minutes.
3. Add salt and pepper to taste.

Nutritional Information:

- Calories-93g
- Fat-6.6g
- Carbs-7.5g
- Protein-1.1g

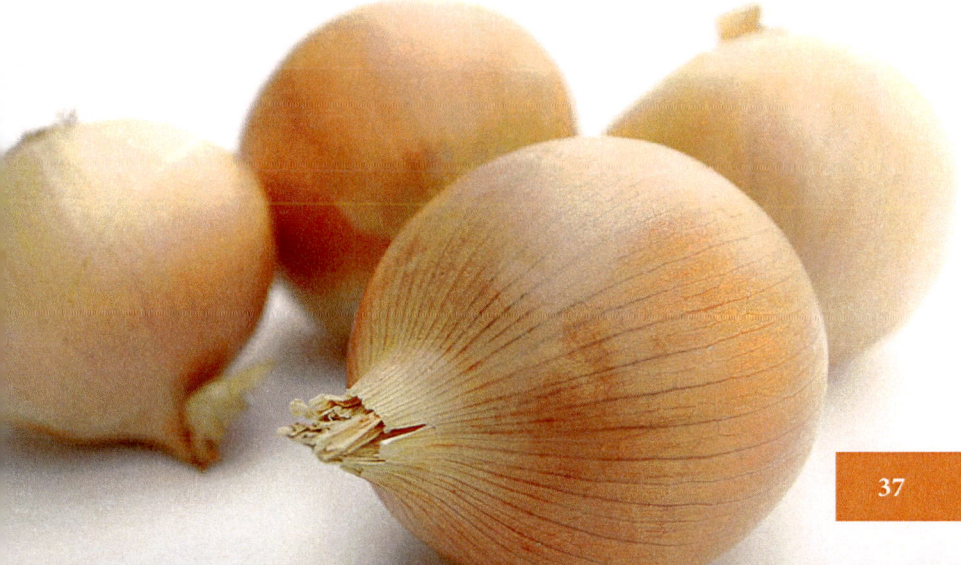

Bacon Smothered Beef

Ingredients:

- Raw ground beef, 6 ounces
- 1 Green onion
- Bacon, 3 slices
- Water, ½ cup
- Heavy cream or coconut milk, ¼ cup
- Pinch of salt and pepper

Preparation:

1. Form a meat patty with the ground beef, brown in a skillet, and set aside.
2. Using the same pan, cook the bacon and then drain and set aside.
3. Place green onion in the same pan.
4. Reduce heat then add water and coconut cream.
5. Stir occasionally while cooking until the onion becomes soft. Add thickening agent if desired.
6. Add the bacon, salt, pepper, to the onion/cream mixture and pour over the meat before serving.

Nutritional Information:

- Calories-633
- Fat-50.5g
- Carbs-3.8g
- Protein-39.8g
- Sodium-1055mg
- Potassium-586mg

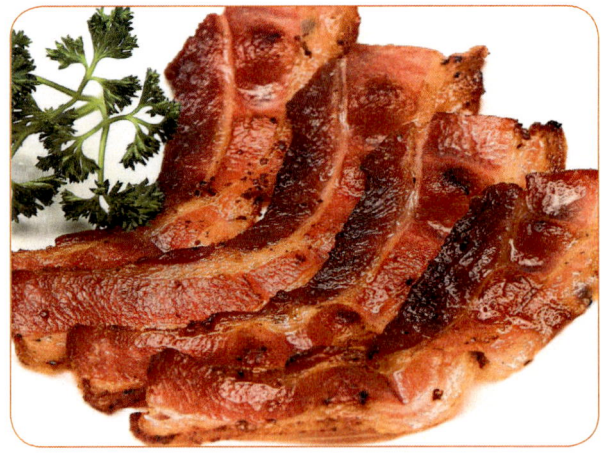

Smoked Eggs Peek-a-Boo

Ingredients:

- 2 large eggs
- Smoked Gouda cheese, 1 ounce – grated or sliced
- Bacon, 4 slices

Preparation:

1. Preheat oven to 350 degrees.
2. Cook bacon until halfway done.
3. Top with Gouda cheese in a way that creates a little depression on each side.
4. Crack the eggs gently into the depressions.
5. Bake in a 350-degree oven for 10 minutes.

Nutritional Information:

- Calories-227g
- Fat-18g
- Carbs-1.1g
- Protein-15.2g
- Sodium-633g
- Potassium-157g

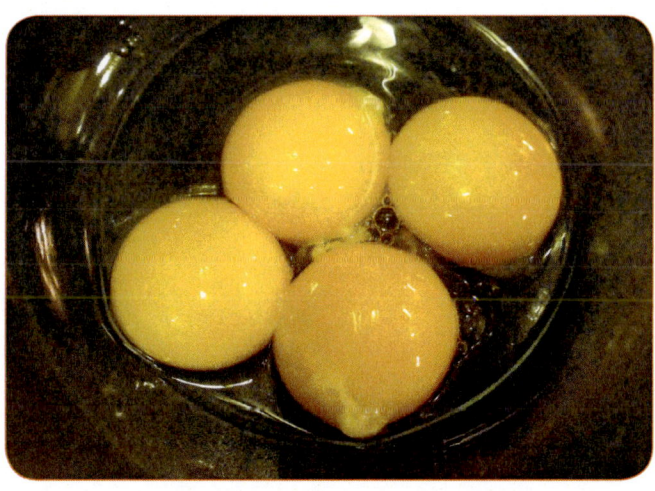

Creamy Leek and Bacon Soup

Ingredients:

- Low-sodium bacon, 5 slices
- 2 Leeks – washed well, sliced thinly
- Water, 2 cups
- Homemade chicken broth, 2 cups
- Heavy cream, 2 cups
- Salt and pepper

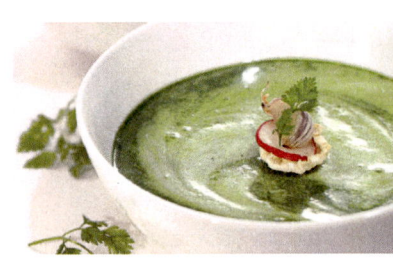

Preparation:

1. Start by browning bacon in a large soup pot.
2. When done, add sliced leeks.
3. Sauté for a few minutes while stirring frequently.
4. Lower heat and simmer for 5-10 minutes.
5. Add cream and bring to a boil.
6. Simmer for a few more minutes and allow thickening.
7. Serve with your favorite vegetables.

Nutritional Information:

- Calories-377
- Fat-37g
- Carbs-5.58g
- Protein-6.1g
- Sodium-211mg
- Potassium-216mg

Chipotle-Lime, Shrimp-Topped Fish

Ingredients:

- 2 Fish filets – 6 ounces each
- 8 Shrimp – medium sized & de-veined
- Onion, 2 ounces – chopped
- Garlic, 2 cloves – minced
- Pork sausage, 3 ounces – crumbled
- 1 Jalapeno – seeded and chopped
- 1 Chipotle pepper (2")
- Juice of 1 lime
- Tequila, 3 tablespoons
- Marmalade, 2 tablespoons
- Homemade seafood stock, ¾ cup
- Pinch of Spanish paprika
- Dash of salt
- Butter, 3 tablespoons

Preparation:

1. Melt the butter in a non-stick pan.
2. Dip fish fillets in melted better.
3. Coat the shrimp and arrange around buttered fish fillets.
4. Sprinkle ½ of the chopped jalapeno over the shrimp.
5. Sprinkle the seafood blend over the exposed side of fish and shrimp.
6. Set aside until sauce starts to simmer.
7. Using the same skillet over medium-high heat, melt the rest of the butter.
8. Butter and brown the sausages.
9. Add in onions, garlic, and salt, and sauté until the onion is tender.
10. Add the remaining jalapeno, paprika, and chipotle.
11. Next add lime marmalade, tequila, and chicken or seafood stock.
12. Reduce heat to its lowest setting until the volume of liquid is reduced by half.
13. Place the pan with the seafood under the pre-heated broiler while the sauce simmers.
14. The fish is done as soon as it becomes opaque. Be careful not to overcook! Remove from pan and either place on individual plates or on one large serving platter.
15. Drizzle sauce over fish then top with shrimp.

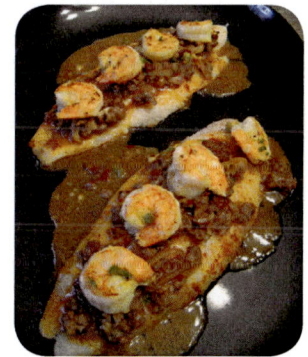

Nutritional Information:

- Calories-448
- Fat-32g
- Carbs-6.8g
- Protein-22.5g
- Sodium-530mg
- Potassium-365mg

Spanish Stewed Beef

Ingredients:

- 1 Carrot, medium-sized – cubed
- Beef, 1½ pounds boneless – cooked and cut into cubes
- Water, 3 cups or just enough to cover beef
- 1 Green bell pepper, medium sized – sliced and seeded
- Onion, 5 ounces – sliced or chopped
- 1 Jalapeno pepper – sliced
- Pimiento, ¼ cup – sliced
- Garlic, 1 clove – minced
- 5 Roma tomatoes – chopped
- 1 Bay leaf
- Extra-virgin olive oil, 2 tablespoons
- Ground cloves, 1/8 teaspoon
- Salt, black pepper, and cinnamon to taste

Preparation:

1. Place cut-up meat in pressure cooker and cover with water.
2. Add in carrots and bring to a boil.
3. Allow to simmer in low heat for 45 minutes to 1 hour after boiling.
4. Remove cover and add the rest of the ingredients.
5. Replace lid and allow to boil for another 20 minutes or until the vegetables are tender.
6. Release pressure and add your favorite thickener.
7. Serve over a bed of rice or pasta.

Nutritional Information:

- Calories-306
- Fat-11.8g
- Carbs-6.83g
- Fiber-1.7g
- Protein-40.42g
- Sodium-186mg
- Potassium-441mg

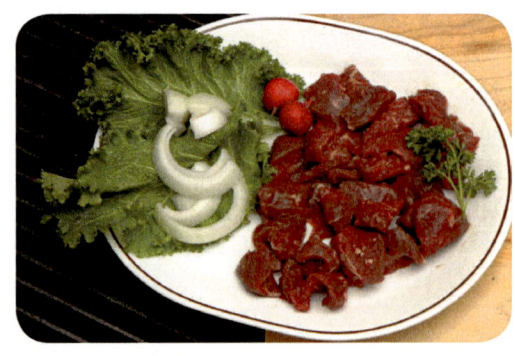

Swiss Steak

Ingredients:

- Resistant Wheat starch, 1 tablespoon
- Beef cube steak, 16 ounces
- Onion, 4 ounces – sliced
- Coconut oil, 2 tablespoons
- 3 Roma tomatoes – cubed
- 1 Green red bell pepper, large
- Water, 2 cups
- Red wine, ¼ cup
- Small amount of your favorite thickener

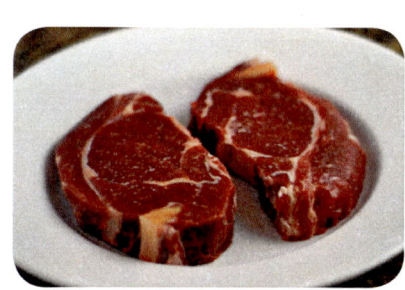

Preparation:

1. Divide the meat into 4 portions.
2. Pound on both sides to tenderize.
3. Dredge with resistant wheat starch.
4. Allow to brown on both sides over high heat in a non-stick skillet.
5. Add onion and brown for a minute or two longer.
6. Next add bell pepper, tomato, wine, and water.
7. Reduce heat to simmer to allow the meat to tenderize, but do not let the veggies get too soft.
8. Add thickener as desired.
9. Serve topped with veggies and spices, or with a side of mashed cauliflower or zucchini noodles.

Nutritional Information:

- Calories-352.3g
- Fat-15.75g
- Carbs-8.3
- Protein-40g
- Sodium-97mg
- Potassium-530mg

Pepper Jack Stromboli

Ingredients:

- 1 slice of focaccia bread
- Lean deli ham, 1 ounce
- Pepper jack cheese, 2 slices
- Hard salami, 1 thin slice
- 2-3 Black olives – sliced

Preparation:

1. Slice the bread into two thin pieces.
2. Place the pepper jack cheese slice on one side of the bread.
3. Add the ham and salami then top with another slice of cheese.
4. Cover with olives then top with the remaining piece of bread.
5. Microwave just until the cheese melts.

Nutritional Information:

- Calories-474
- Fat-38g
- Carbs-8.6g
- Protein-29.6g
- Sodium-1100mg

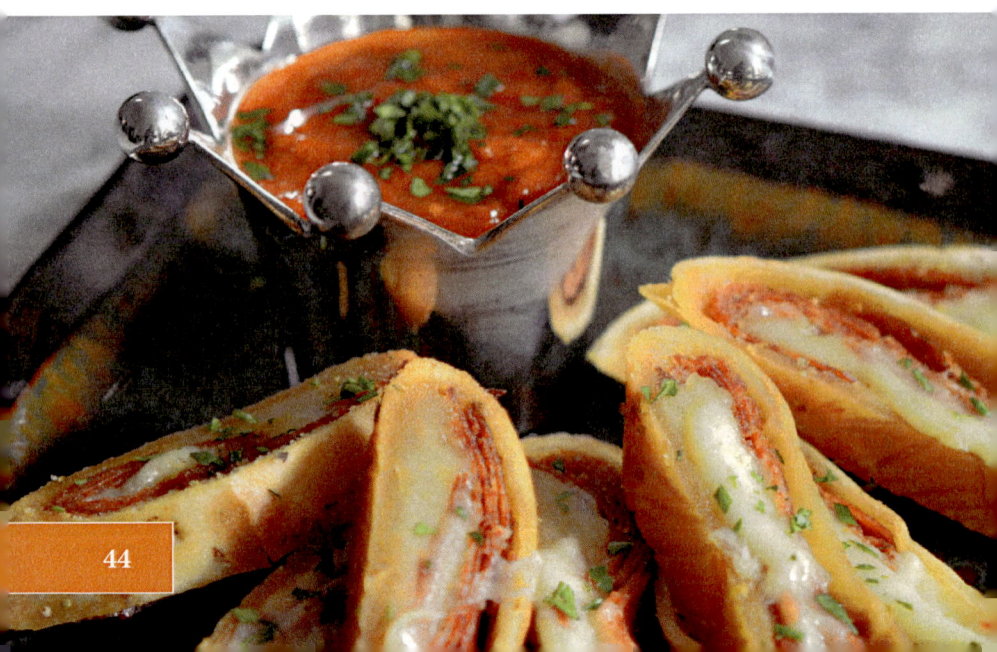

Homemade Chicken Lettuce Wrap

Ingredients:

- Mayonnaise, 4 tablespoons
- Romaine lettuce leaves, 2 large pieces
- 6 Roma tomatoes
- Chicken meat, 4 ounces – baked or charbroiled
- Olive oil, 2 teaspoons
- Onion, 1 ounce – slivered
- Dash of salt

Preparation:

1. Sauté onion in olive oil until it caramelizes and turns brown.
2. Turn off heat and add the mayo.
3. Place lettuce leaves on plates the lay chicken on lettuce bed.
4. Next add mayo mixture on chicken.
5. Top with tomato slices, roll up lettuce with ingredients inside then enjoy with your favorite spices.

Nutritional Information:

- Calories-363
- Fat-32.1g
- Carbs-2.82g
- Protein-16.5g
- Sodium-320mg

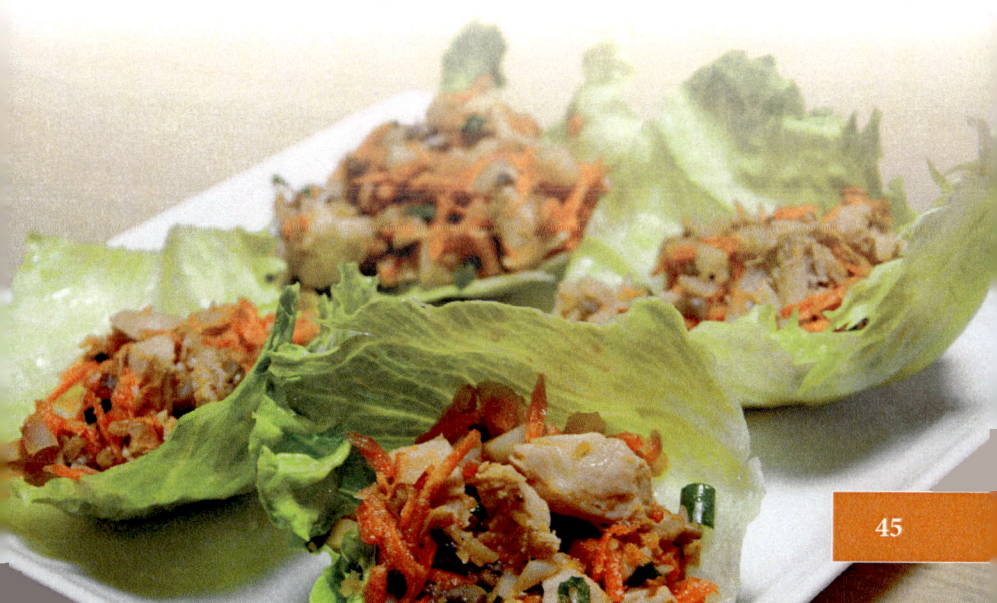

Sausage Tortilla Casserole

Ingredients:

- Lean ground pork or pork sausage, 8 ounces
- Yellow squash, 5 ounces – diced
- 1 Leek – sliced lengthwise
- Cilantro, 3 sprigs – chopped
- Red bell pepper, ¼ cup – diced
- 1 Corn tortilla – crumbled to pieces
- Cheddar cheese, 6 ounces – grated
- Sprinkle of chili powder

Preparation:

1. Preheat oven to 350 degrees.
2. Brown sausage or ground pork in hot skillet until no longer pink.
3. Add squash and red pepper then sauté for a few minutes while stirring continuously.
4. Add leeks and continue cooking until all veggies are just done.
5. Add the cilantro, tortilla, and chili powder.
6. Pour everything into greased baking dish and top with cheese.
7. Bake for 20 minutes or until the cheese is melted. It can be served with guacamole salad on the side.

Nutritional Information:

- Calories-414
- Fat-30.1g
- Carbs-12.53g
- Protein-24.4
- Potassium-540mg
- Sodium-570mg

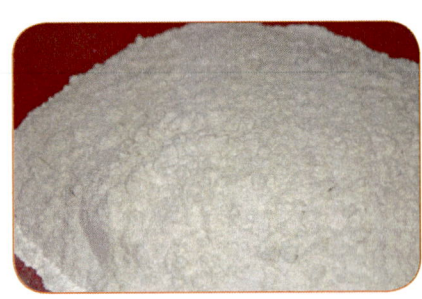

Meatballs and Kale Soup

Ingredients:

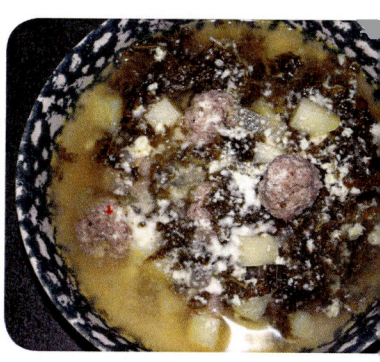

- McCormick Montreal seasoning, 1 tablespoon
- Lean ground pork, 1 pound
- Onion, 3 ounces – sliced
- Clarified butter or olive oil, 2 tablespoons
- Homemade chicken broth, 7 cups
- Cauliflower, ½ cup – cooked and mashed
- Kale leaves, 2 cups – chopped
- 1 Carrot – peeled and sliced thin
- Ground chia seeds, 1 teaspoon
- Black pepper to taste

Preparation:

1. Rub the seasoning into the ground pork.
2. Heat oil or butter in a large soup pot.
3. Add onions and sauté until it begins to caramelize.
4. Add broth and carrot then bring to a boil.
5. Using a spoon, form small meatballs with the pork and drop gently into the broth.
6. When the broth simmers, lower the heat.
7. Add in the chia seeds and mashed cauliflower.
8. Flavor with black pepper to taste. Serve with your favorite crackers.

Nutritional Information:

- Calories-351
- Fat-24g
- Carbs-5.73g
- Fiber-1.23g
- Protein-21g
- Sodium-439mg
- Potassium-704mg

Hotdog Goulash

Ingredients:

- Sugar-free bacon, 2 slices – chopped
- Onions, 2 ounces – sliced
- 1 Sugar-free uncured hotdog – sliced
- Mayonnaise, 3 tablespoons
- **Shawarma spice blend:**
- Ground cumin seed, 2 tablespoons
- Turmeric, 2 tablespoons
- Ground coriander seed, 2 tablespoons
- Garlic powder, 2 teaspoons
- Onion powder, 1 teaspoon
- Cayenne, 1 teaspoon

Preparation:

1. Mix all the spices together and store in an airtight container until ready for use.
2. Heat a non-stick skillet and cook bacon until crisp.
3. Add onion and cook until tender.
4. Next add hotdog slices and cook mixture for a couple of minutes.
5. Add the broccoli and continue cooking while stirring until the vegetables just turn tender.
6. Turn off heat before adding Shawarma spice blend and mayo.
7. Stir to blend in the sauce then serve.

Nutritional Information:

- Calories-537
- Fat-48.6
- Carbs-12.5g
- Protein-17.5g
- Sodium-845mg
- Potassium-415mg

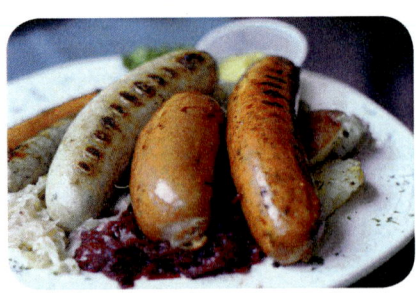

Pork and Broccoli Stir-Fry With Kelp Noodles

Ingredients:

- Olive oil, 2 tablespoons
- Red palm oil, 1 teaspoon
- Lean pork, 4 ounces – cut into thin strips
- Onion, 2 ounces – slivered
- Bell pepper, 2 ounces – sliced
- Broccoli florets, 1/2 cup
- Garlic, 1 clove – minced
- Fresh ginger, ½ teaspoon
- Chili paste, ¼ teaspoon
- Homemade chicken broth, ½ cup
- Coconut aminos, 1 teaspoon
- Sesame seeds, 3 teaspoons
- Kelp noodles, 8 ounces
- Pinch of dehydrated onion
- Pinch of your preferred thickener

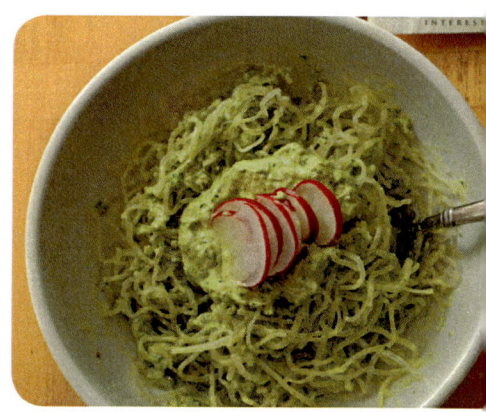

Preparation:

1. Heat oil in a non-stick skillet over high heat.
2. Add meat and stir-fry until brown.
3. Add onion and bell pepper and sauté just until tender.
4. Add the rest of the ingredients except for the thickener. (If necessary, thicken before topping noodles with sauce.)
5. Meanwhile, rinse the kelp noodles in a colander under hot water.
6. Drain noodles then add meat toppings and serve hot.

Nutritional Information:

- Calories-230
- Fat-15mg
- Carbs-9.05g
- Fiber-2.95g
- Protein-15g
- Sodium-225mg
- Potassium-478mg

10 Recipes for Dinner

Smothered Pork Chops

Ingredients:

- Lean pork loin, 10 ounces
- Bacon, 2 ounces – coarsely chopped
- Onions, 2 ounces – slivered in long strips
- 4 Mushrooms, large
- Chicken broth, 1 cup
- Heavy cream, 2 ounces
- White wine, 1 ounce
- Dash of salt and pepper

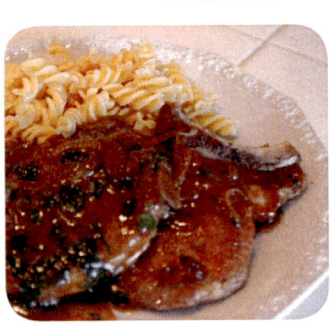

Preparation:

1. Preheat oven to 350 degrees.
2. Brown bacon in a non-stick skillet over high heat.
3. Add in mushroom slices and continue to sauté just until they are no longer white, then remove and set aside.
4. Brown the meat on all sides in the same skillet.
5. Add the vegetable mixture back into the pan along with chicken broth, pepper, and wine.
6. Remove from heat and cover before placing in the oven.
7. Allow to cook for about 30 minutes.
8. Remove from oven and add cream.
9. Allow to simmer over low heat on the stovetop.
10. Serve with your favorite veggies or salad.

Nutritional Information:

- Calories- 475g
- Fat-32g
- Carbs-5.55g
- Fiber-1.2g
- Protein-37mg
- Sodium-593mg
- Potassium-909mg

Mushroom Barley Soup

Ingredients:

- 1 large pork or beef bone
- Onion, 3 ounces – chopped
- Celery, 1 cup – chopped
- Fresh mushrooms, 12 ounces
- Beef or pork broth, 1 cup
- Water, 1½ quarts
- Pearl barley, ¼ cup
- Salt, ¼ teaspoon
- Black pepper, ¼ teaspoon
- Onion powder, ¼ teaspoon
- Heavy cream, 1 cup
- Sprinkle of cayenne or paprika

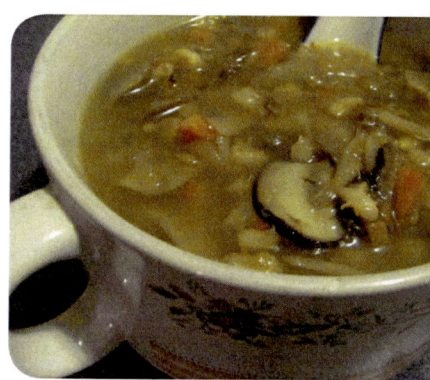

Preparation:

1. Place the bone in a pressure cooker.
2. Add in everything except for the last cream, cayenne, and/or paprika.
3. Seal the lid and cook under pressure for 8-10 minutes.
4. As soon as the knob starts to rock gently, cook for an additional 20 minutes at reduced heat.
5. Remove cooker from heat and run cold water over it while the pressure is being released.
6. Add in the cream and a thickener if desired.
7. Continue to cook until you get the preferred consistency.
8. Serve with low-carb crackers or bread.

Nutritional Information:

- Calories-292
- Fat-16.05g
- Carbs-12.22g
- Fiber-9.54g
- Protein-24.88g
- Sodium443mg
- Potassium-659mg

Italian Cottage Pie

Ingredients:

- Lean ground beef, 1 pound
- Italian sausage, 8 ounces
- Green bell pepper, 1 cup
- Onion, 2 ounces – chopped
- Garlic, 2 cloves – minced
- Tomatoes, 1 can – diced
- Black pepper, ¼ teaspoon
- Dash of pepper
- Dried oregano, ¼ teaspoon
- Steamed cauliflower, 2 cups
- Cheddar cheese, 8 ounces – grated

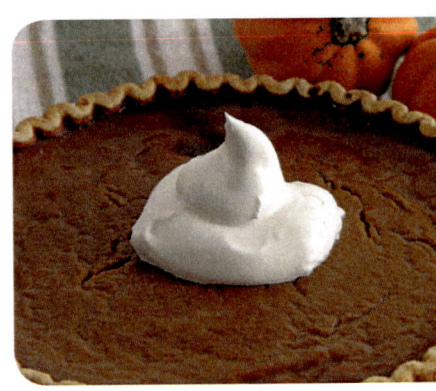

Preparation:

1. Cook cauliflower any way you like until just about tender.
2. Brown the crumbled beef and Italian sausage in a skillet over medium-high heat.
3. Add in onion and green pepper then sauté until onion is translucent.
4. Add in tomatoes, garlic, salt, pepper, and oregano.
5. Preheat oven to 350 degrees.
6. Simmer meat mixture until the tomatoes are tender enough to start falling apart.
7. Drain any liquid off the cauliflower and mash with butter and cream.
8. Spread cauliflower over the meat mixture.
9. Top with cheese and bake for 30 minutes then serve with your salad of choice.

Nutritional Information:

- Calories-468
- Carbs-8.42g
- Fat-31.9g
- Fiber-6.24g
- Protein-35g
- Potassium-428mg
- Sodium-726mg

Rosemary Pork Shoulder Rest

Ingredients:

- Pork, 7 pound-"picnic"-shoulder roast
- Onion powder, ½ teaspoon
- Rosemary, 1 tablespoon freshly chopped
- Dash of salt and pepper

Preparation:

1. Preheat oven to 350 degrees.
2. Place roast in a baking pan and sprinkle salt, pepper, onion powder, and rosemary.
3. Place in the oven and cook for 30-40 minutes per pound.
4. Slice and serve with drippings.

Nutritional Information:

- Calories-260
- Fat-14.3g
- Carbs-0.3g
- Protein-30.3g
- Sodium-246mg
- Potassium-402mg

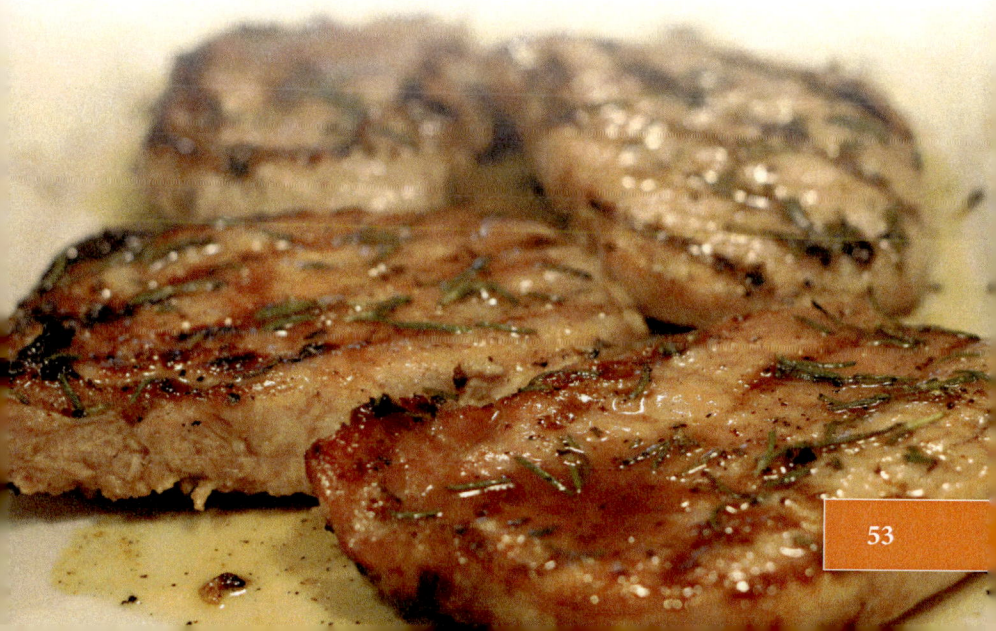

Asian Pork and Cabbage

Ingredients:

- Pork loin or ground pork, 12 ounces
- Green cabbage, 2 cups – sliced
- Red bell pepper, 1/3 cup
- 3 Green onions – chopped
- 4 Mushrooms, large – sliced
- Ginger, ½ teaspoon – minced
- Garlic, 2 cloves – minced
- Chili paste, 1 teaspoon
- Soy sauce, 1 tablespoon
- Low-sodium chicken broth, 1 cup
- Coconut oil or oil of your choice, 3 tablespoons

Preparation:

1. Sauté mushroom with oil in a large wok over high heat until halfway done.
2. Add meat and stir-fry until no longer visibly pink.
3. Add seasonings and veggies.
4. Continue to sauté until cabbage is soft.
5. Add in liquid ingredients and simmer for 2-3 minutes then serve immediately.

Nutritional Information:

- Calories-304
- Fat-18.7g
- Carbs-6.88g
- Fiber-2.15g
- Protein-26.8mg
- Sodium-510mg
- Potassium-605mg

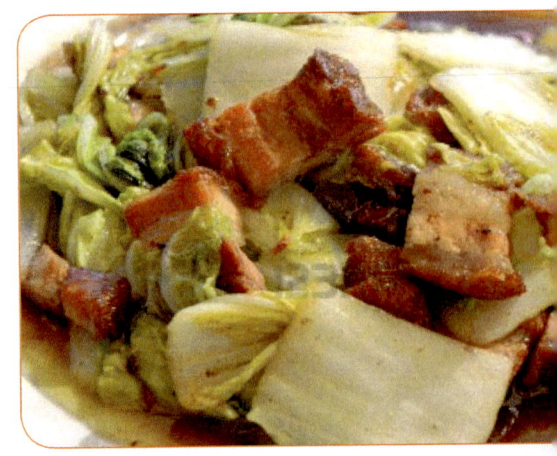

Asian Fish Soup

Ingredients:

- Coconut oil, 1 tablespoon + Red palm oil, 1 teaspoon
- Green onion, ½ cup – chopped
- 5 Red radishes – sliced
- Homemade chicken stock, 2½ cups
- Coconut cream, 4 ounces
- Fish sauce, 2 tablespoons
- Sambal olek chili paste, ½ teaspoon
- Turmeric, ½ teaspoon
- Ground coriander, ½ teaspoon
- Ginger root, 1 teaspoon – minced
- Garlic, 1 clove – minced
- Yam shirataki noodles, one 8-ounce bag
- Fresh cilantro, ½ cup – chopped
- 1 Medium banana – sliced into chunks
- Fish filets, 1 pound – sliced into chunks

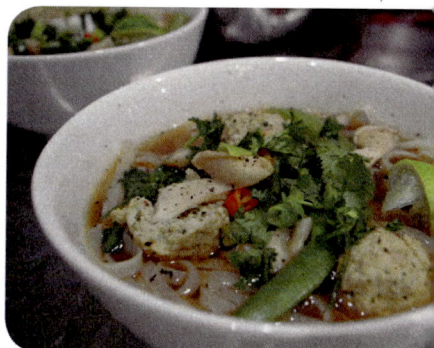

Preparation:

1. Melt oil in a large saucepot.
2. Add radishes and sliced onion.
3. Add the remaining ingredients except banana and noodles.
4. Simmer until radish is tender … about 10 minutes.
5. Add bananas and fish to soup pot.
6. Simmer.
7. Serve with blanched and rinsed noodles.

Nutritional Information:

- Calories-233
- Fat-20g
- Carbs-8.32g
- Fiber-1.48g
- Protein-14.7g
- Sodium-586mg
- Potassium-275mg

Salmon in Creamy Bacon Sauce

Ingredients:

- Unsalted butter, 1 tablespoon
- Salmon, 2 filets
- Bacon, 3 slices – chopped
- Green onion, ½ cup – chopped
- Coconut cream, ¼ cup + 2 tablespoons
- Mayonnaise, ¼ cup + 2 tablespoons
- Shawarma blend, ½ teaspoon
- **Shawarma spice blend:**
- Ground cumin seed, 2 tablespoons
- Turmeric, 2 tablespoons
- Ground coriander seed, 2 tablespoons
- Garlic powder, 2 teaspoons
- Onion powder, 1 teaspoons
- Cayenne, 1 teaspoon

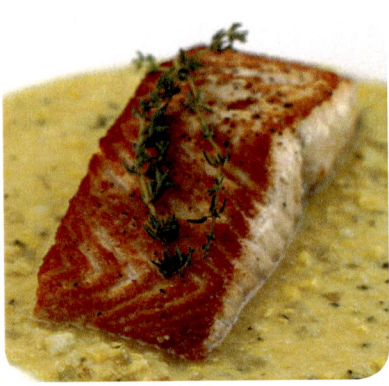

Preparation:

1. Mix all the spices together and store in an airtight container until ready for use.
2. Melt butter in a dish and then coat salmon fillets with it on each side.
3. Broil for about 5 minutes on both sides until firm in the center.
4. While fish is cooking, brown bacon in a non-stick skillet over high-heat.
5. Reduce heat then add green onion.
6. While on the lowest heat, add coconut cream, spice blend, and stir.
7. Turn off the heat.
8. When fish is done, place on serving plates.
9. Add mayo to the skillet and stir just long enough to blend.
10. Immediately pour half the sauce on each filet.

Nutritional Information:

- Calories-706
- Fat-799g
- Carbs-2.6g
- Fiber-1.8g
- Protein-5.3g
- Sodium-280mg
- Potassium-135mg

Tilapia in Shawarma Sauce

Ingredients:

- Tilapia filets, four 5-ounce servings
- Unsalted butter, 2 tablespoons
- 1 ½ teaspoon Shawarma blend
- Homemade mayo, 1/3 cup
- Heavy cream or coconut milk, 2 tablespoons
- **Shawarma spice blend:**
- Ground cumin seed, 2 tablespoons
- Turmeric, 2 tablespoons
- Ground coriander seed, 2 tablespoons
- Garlic powder, 2 teaspoons
- Onion powder, 1 teaspoon
- Cayenne, 1 teaspoon

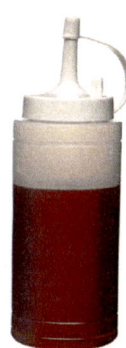

Preparation:

1. Mix all the spices together and store in an airtight container until ready for use.
2. Combine spice blend, cream or coconut milk, and mayo in a small serving dish.
3. In the meantime, sauté the fish in melted butter in a non-stick skillet over medium-high heat.
4. Remove the moisture off the fish by lightly dabbing with a paper towel.
5. Sprinkle both sides evenly with the remaining ½ teaspoon and a pinch of salt.
6. Raise the heat to high and sear the fish on both sides until golden brown and cooked in the center.
7. Plate the fillets and spoon about 2 tablespoon of sauce over each.
8. Serve with a green vegetables or a salad.

Nutritional Information:

- Calories-338.5
- Fat-25g
- Carbs-0.63g
- Fiber 0.13g
- Protein-28.3g
- Sodium-83mg
- Potassium-435mg

Middle–Eastern Baked Fish

Ingredients:

- Caraway seed, ½ teaspoon
- Cumin seed, ½ teaspoon
- Coriander seed, ½ teaspoon
- Red pepper flakes, ¼ teaspoon
- Onion powder, ½ teaspoon
- Onion, 3 ounces – thinly sliced
- Unsalted butter, 2 tablespoons
- Garlic, 2 large cloves
- Parsley, 2 tablespoons – finely minced
- Mild fish filets, 24 ounces
- Tomato paste, 1 tablespoons

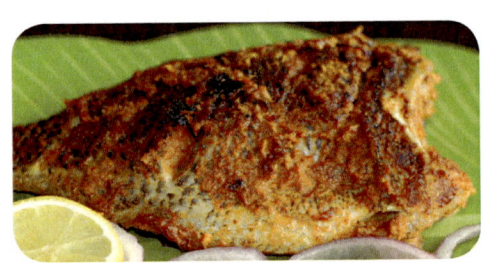

Preparation:

1. Preheat oven to 350 degrees.
2. Place the first 4 spices listed in a skillet over dry heat until fragrant.
3. Remove and place into a coffee grinder and grind over medium-fire then set aside.
4. Place the fish fillets in the pan and allow to cook, then remove from pan.
5. In the same skillet, melt the butter then add onions and brown slightly over medium heat.
6. Add garlic then sprinkle half of the previously toasted spices and parsley over the onions/butter.
7. Lay the fillets evenly over the onion mixture.
8. Spread the tomato paste on the fillets and sprinkle with the remaining garlic, butter, and onion mixture.
9. Place in the oven and bake for 20 minutes then serve with your favorite salad.

Nutritional Information:

- Calories-176
- Fat-9.8g
- Carbs-4.3g
- Fiber-0.98g

- Protein-20.4g
- Sodium-70mg
- Potassium-124mg

Squash-Pumpkin Soup

Ingredients:

- Lean bacon, 4 ounces – chopped
- Yellow summer squash, 1 cup – sliced small
- Pumpkin puree, ½ cup
- Purple or white onions, 2 ounces – cooked with squash
- Homemade chicken stock, 2 cups
- Coconut milk, ¾ cup
- Coarse black pepper, ¼ teaspoon

Preparation:

1. Brown bacon in a non-stick skillet until crisp.
2. Remove from pan and set aside.
3. Add squash and onion to the same pan and continue to sauté until squash is completely cooked.
4. Place this mixture into a food processor and pulse until smooth.
5. Return to skillet.
6. Add the rest of the ingredients including the cooked bacon.
7. Simmer until thick and serve hot.

Nutritional Information:

- Calories-388
- Fat-33.5g
- Carbs 9.67g
- Fiber-6.54g
- Protein-11.2g
- Sodium-336mg
- Potassium-595mg

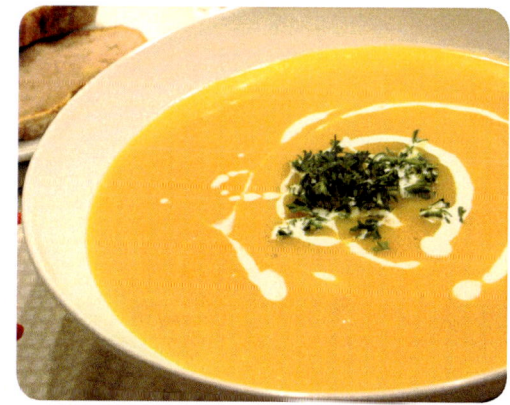

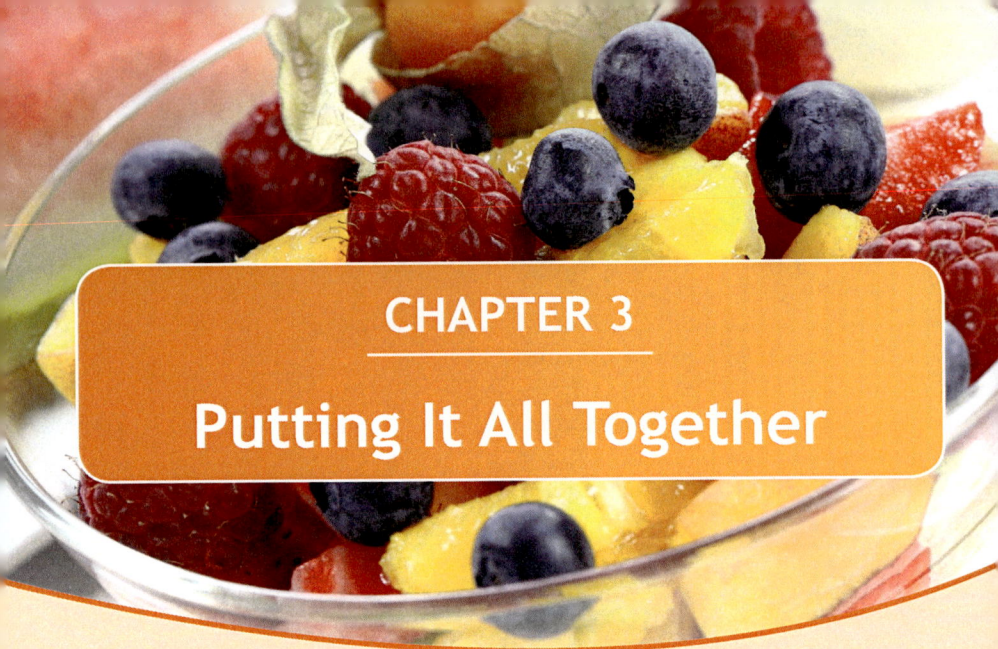

CHAPTER 3

Putting It All Together

Now that you've gained the basic knowledge of how to eat according to the Atkins diet, and also have recipes that you can make easily at home, it is now time for you to make a comprehensive plan in order to rotate your meals properly.

Sample Templates

Preparing Yourself

The first step is for you to have the right mindset. Answer the following questions on a piece of paper and go on your own "self-awareness retreat" to help you set the right goals in making this diet plan work. Take the time to get ready to make these healthy changes in your life and then commit to them.

1. *What is your current diet composed of?*
2. *What are your ideal outcomes for undergoing the Atkins Diet?*
3. *What are the health concerns that you want to address throughout this program?*
4. *How will this program benefit you?*
5. *What are the things you can do to help yourself both commit and succeed with this diet plan?*

Your Daily Motivational Guide

Finish these statements daily to help keep your motivation at its peak:

1. *Today I will keep myself healthy by sticking to the Atkins diet. In order to do this, I will: …*
2. *I am doing this for my health because I want to …*

Your Atkins Diet Plan

Date	Breakfast	Lunch	Dinner
Monday			
Tuesday			
Wednesday			
Thursday			
Friday			
Saturday			
Sunday			

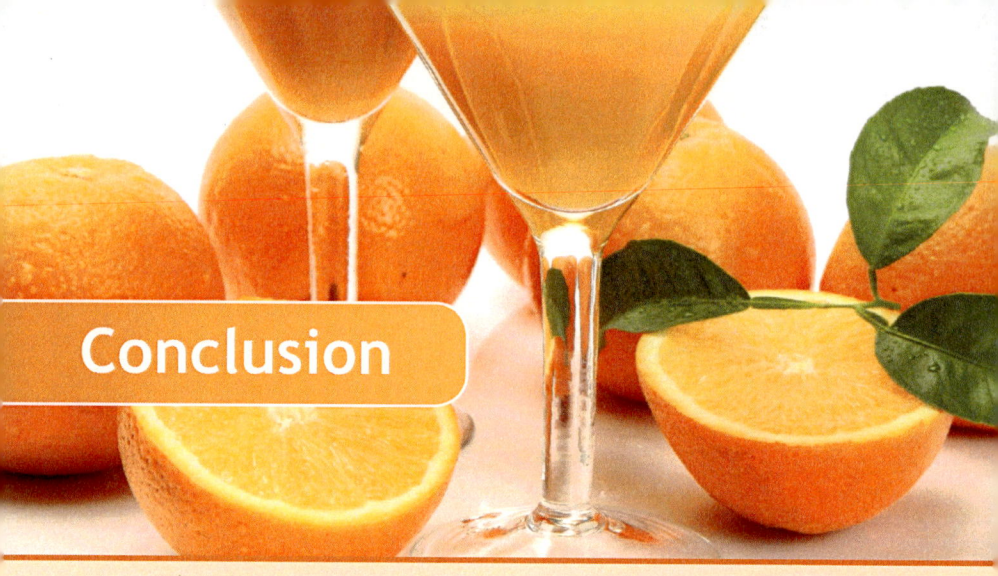

Conclusion

Now that you've reached the end of the program, and hopefully your goal weight, don't stop now! We're sure that with the help of this guide and your own motivations, you've successfully completed the Atkins diet program. We are confident that you are now on the lifelong maintenance phase, and living a healthier life.

While it may be tempting to succumb every now and then, learning to exercise self-control and discipline is a skill that can be learned over time. Don't be too hard on yourself when you do sneak a cupcake, but remember to compensate for these occasional treats.

It's a good idea to keep your personal food triggers out of your home or workplace. They can trigger cravings that you don't need . There's nothing wrong with indulging once in a while, but remember to always keep it in moderation. When you've had a bad carb day, don't give up. Try to do better the next day. In time, you will get used to your usual low carb diet, and you will soon find that you barely even miss eating carbohydrates!

The Atkins diet is a wonderful way of letting you experience a whole new reality of a healthy lifestyle. You will feel better, healthier, happier, and have a hunger for life instead of carbs! So make this pact with us … take our hand … and let us help you get healthier with the Atkins Diet!

Oh, and remember to claim your special bonus of *10 Healthy Dinner Recipes* by clicking here: http://www.expertsfeatured.com/jennifer-bonus-recipes/

-- Jennifer Jenkins